Daventry

perfect
bride

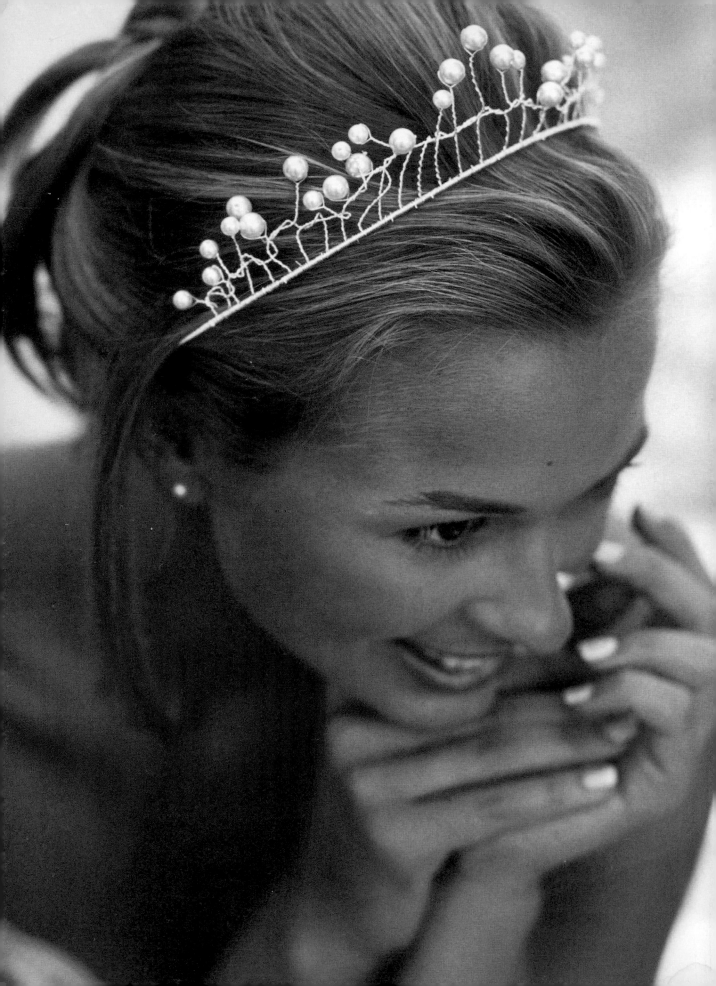

perfect bride

Janet Wright

hamlyn

First published in Great Britain in
2005 by Hamlyn, a division of
Octopus Publishing Group Ltd,
2–4 Heron Quays, London E14 4JP

Copyright © Octopus Publishing
Group Ltd 2005

Distributed in the United States
and Canada by
Sterling Publishing Co., Inc.
387 Park Avenue South, New
York, NY 10016-8810

Wedding™ is a trademark of
IPC Media, copyright IPC
Media Limited 2005

The moral rights of the author
have been asserted.

ISBN 0 600 61244 9
EAN 980600612445

A CIP catalogue record for this
book is available from the British
Library

Printed and bound in China
10 9 8 7 6 5 4 3 2 1

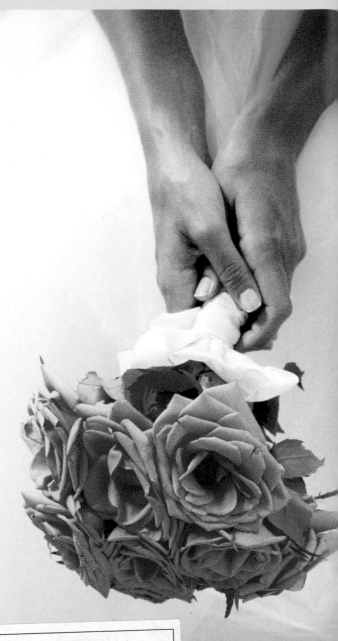

contents

how to use this book

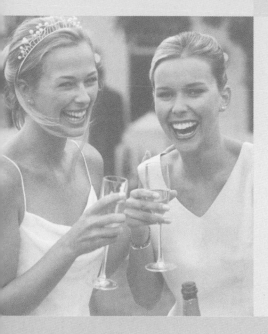

Congratulations on your forthcoming wedding, and your wise decision to get organized in advance, be it six months or six weeks ahead. Full of exercises, healthy eating and beauty tips, this book will help you stay on top of the planning and shape up to look your best on the big day. Be realistic about your goals. Unless you're heavily overweight, don't aim to lose more than two dress sizes – you could set yourself up to fail and feel bad when you should be celebrating. Focus on the many other techniques in this book to enhance your natural assets.

read ahead

Before you begin each section, read through the exercises and imagine yourself carrying out the programme. This will help you both to do the exercises and to stick with the routine. You should also read the final week's section (see pages 82–101) well in advance. Check that you've already tried anything you'll be doing that week, apart from simple treatments such as massages. Don't do anything new in the final week, or use any untested products, in case of a skin reaction.

Some parts of this book need to be followed in the order in which they appear – aerobic exercise before muscle building, for example, and facial exercises started early enough to show an effect – but many can be tried out at any time. Try the detox from the 6-week Fit Bride Plan (see page 110) if you're feeling sluggish, and the stress-relieving massages from the final week's section as soon as you like. The 6-week Fit Bride Plan is a quick fix for those with limited time. The diet is more stringent and the exercise regime more concentrated, but it is safe to follow indefinitely. Beauty tips can be found in the rest of the book.

and finally...

Please use this book as a resource – not as a source of extra stress! You don't have to follow every suggestion. Remember that everyone thinks the bride looks beautiful and anything that goes wrong at a wedding makes a funny story later on. Above all, your wedding should be a celebration, not an ordeal. Have a wonderful time!

	6 MONTHS	
GOALS	To start long-term preparations and lose weight if necessary	
EXERCISE PLAN	Follow the fat-burning exercise routines on pages 10–19 three or four times a week. On other days, fit in a walk	
EATING PLAN	Choose a good fat-loss food plan following the suggestions on pages 20–25	
BEAUTY PLAN	Bring your skin and hair into top condition. Start treatments that take time to show results	

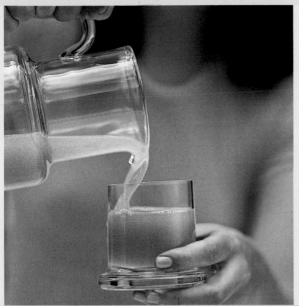
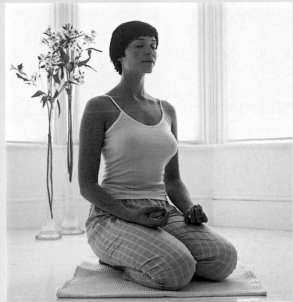

6-month plan at a glance

3 MONTHS	1 MONTH	1 WEEK	WEDDING DAY	6-WEEK FIT BRIDE PLAN
To tackle any problems you've encountered, and home in on the parts you'll be showing off	To deep cleanse and detox, then to create a perfect finish	To ensure a smooth and stress-free run-up to the wedding	To see all your work pay off and enjoy the day	To maximize assets, minimize defects and create the illusion of perfection
Body sculpting for the areas you most need to shape up	Lengthen muscles and boost lymph circulation, while creating a tall, smooth silhouette	Relaxation and stretching	Moving with perfect poise	Fast fat loss and body sculpting
Solve problems with weight or shape	Detox diet for perfect skin, and eating for extra energy	Eat to look and feel your best	Eat to avoid an energy slump	A healthy detox diet to shed extra weight and improve skin tone
Ensure that every-thing revealed by your dress will look perfect	Skin-enhancing treatments and photo-perfect make-up	Pampering and perfecting	Dress for success, and have your emergency repair kit at hand	Focus on the essentials and tricks to make the camera love you (see pages 108–109)

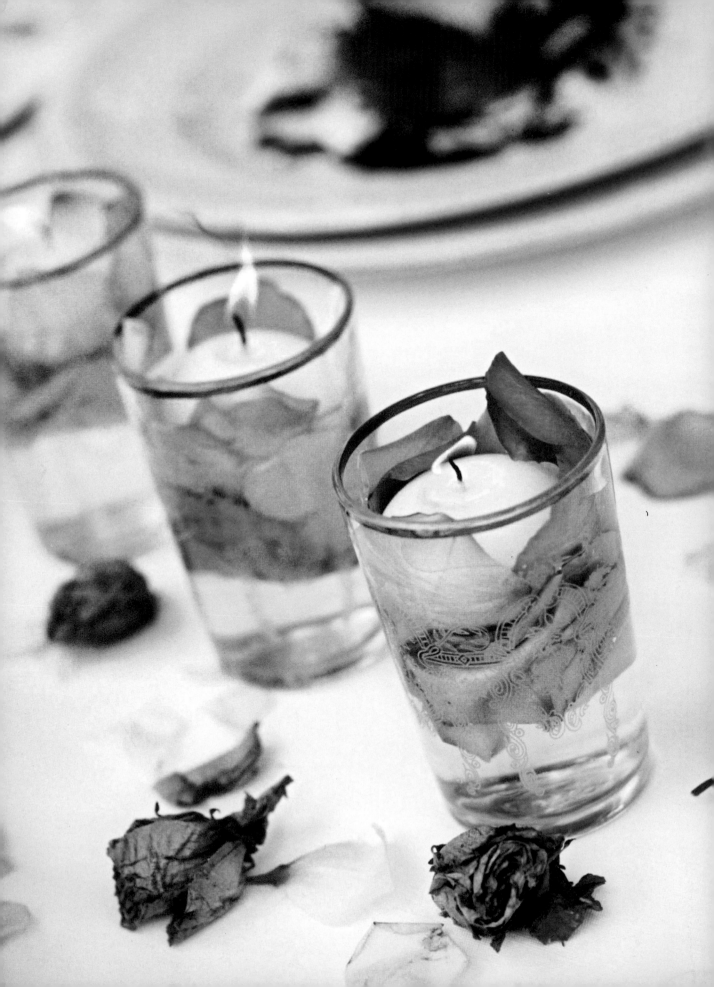

6 months to go

With six months to go before the wedding, you have plenty of time to shape up. A crash diet would leave you weak, stressed-out and haggard. Following **a healthy eating plan** will help you lose any extra weight, with the bonus of better skin, glossy hair and nails that don't split. If you have much weight to lose, you'll see it roll off as you start to eat healthily. But if you're already within a healthy weight range, be prepared for more of an effort.

Create a fit physique by doing fat-burning aerobic exercise. Strengthening your muscles will build shapelier curves and increase your ability to burn fat. Working at this level you're not in danger of looking like Ms Universe – you're toning muscles rather than building bulk.

The final pages of this chapter cover beauty preparations that take time to show results: improving your skin and hair condition, for example. You'll be planning appointments with the dressmaker, hairdresser and beauty salon, but there are also treatments to do at home.

WEDDING PLANNING CHECKLIST: 6–4 MONTHS

You should already have organized most of the following, but if not, do them now:

- Set the date and let everyone know when it is.
- Work out your budget.
- Book the ceremony, venue and caterers.
- Draw up a guest list.
- Choose the best man, ushers and bridesmaids.
- Decide on your theme and colours.
- Order the stationery, including save-the-date cards if you're using them.
- Plan and book your honeymoon, and where you're going to spend the first night.
- Book cars, photographer and videographer.
- Consider taking out wedding insurance.
- Start shopping for rings.
- Book band, DJ and/or musicians to play at your ceremony/reception.
- Choose your own and the bridesmaids' dresses and the men's suits.
- Confirm arrangements with the minister or celebrant, and discuss the service, readings and music.
- Organize your flowers.
- Order the cake.
- Reserve any rented equipment such as cake stand, tables and chairs, marquee and dance flooring.
- Organize your gift list.
- Reserve accommodation for any guests who need it.

fat-burning exercise

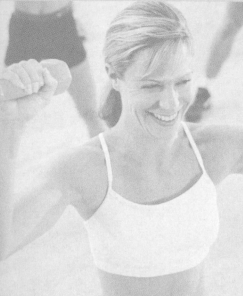

Regular aerobic exercise will burn up fat as well as give you more energy and better skin. Muscle building exercise is valuable, too, as the body uses more calories to maintain muscle than fat. All you need is a watch, a suitable pair of trainers and an optional set of hand weights (see page 39).

When doing the exercises, keep your abdominal muscles ('abs') and pelvic floor muscles engaged, especially when making any movement that could strain your back. In other words, tighten the muscles and hold them firmly, while still breathing normally.

your workout

- First, **warm up** for at least 5 minutes (see below)
- Do **aerobic exercise** for at least 20 minutes (see pages 12–15)
- Slow down gradually over a few minutes, until your heartbeat returns to normal. Then do **muscle building** (see page 16–17)
- Finish with **stretching exercises** for a few minutes (see opposite)

Start by doing 20–30 minutes of aerobic exercise, two or three times a week, followed by up to 10 minutes of muscle building. Build up to an hour of exercise three times a week by the end of the first month.

> **SAFETY FIRST**
> Before starting, check with your doctor to make sure you have no medical condition that would be affected by exercising. Always listen to your body: stop doing anything that hurts, and if pain persists, seek medical advice.

warming up

Always start your exercise session by warming up for at least 5 minutes. Repeat each warm-up exercise five to ten times.

March on the spot March slowly at first, then build up speed, putting your whole foot down each time. Music helps you keep moving, so put on your favourite dance track. Start by marching to every other beat and increase till you're jogging in double time at the end.

Head and shoulders Let your head sink towards each shoulder in turn, then towards your chest. Lift your shoulders towards your ears, drop them, then roll them.

Arm turns Stand with your legs apart and turn, without swinging, to one side and then the other, leading with your outstretched arms. Keep your hips still to prevent your knees twisting.

Pliés Stand with your legs wide apart, your feet turned out and your knees pointing the same way as your feet. Bend your knees deeply, without extending them past your toes or sticking your bottom out.

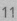

stretching

Finally, after some muscle-building work (see pages 16–17), spend a few minutes stretching. Hold each stretch for at least 10 seconds.

Calf stretch Stand in a lunge position as shown, leaning on your front thigh and pressing the back heel as near the floor as feels comfortable.

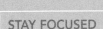

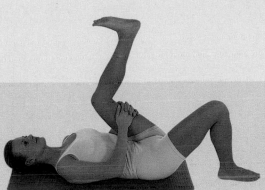

Hamstring stretch Lie on the floor and lift one leg at a time as shown, pulling it gently towards you. Let go and circle the ankle one way and then the other.

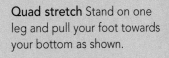

Quad stretch Stand on one leg and pull your foot towards your bottom as shown.

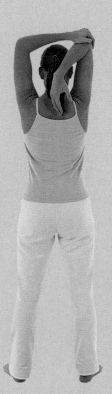

Arm stretch 1 Reach out across your chest to the right with your left arm, gently pushing it in towards your body with the right hand. Repeat on the other side.

Arm stretch 2 Raise your right elbow to the ceiling and reach down behind your shoulder with your right hand; gently increase the stretch by pushing your upper arm backwards with the left hand. Repeat on the other side.

STAY FOCUSED
Pause for a moment to clear your mind and mentally focus on what you're going to do before you start an exercise session. Keep that focus as you work out. Exercising mindfully is more effective, and also relieves stress.

dance the fat away

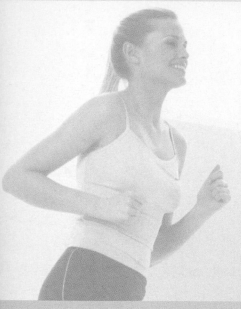

Aerobic exercise is continuous movement at a pace that speeds up your heart rate. You should be breathing harder than normal, still just about able to keep up a conversation. Any kind of aerobic exercise will help you burn fat: brisk walking, dancing, running, skipping, using fitness videos, playing football – anything you like, and the more variety the better. You need to keep going for 20 minutes or more for effective fat burning. As a bonus, your body continues burning fat faster for some time after a workout, so treat yourself to a big healthy breakfast or dinner.

aerobic dance

Put on your favourite energetic dance music and move to the beat. Start with your feet together and return to the start position after each step. Do each movement eight times on each side unless otherwise stated.

Toe taps Tap the toes of your right foot directly in front of you, return to start position, then repeat. After eight times, repeat with the left foot. Then tap your toes in front of the opposite foot, then out to each side.

Heel digs Tap your right heel on the floor in front of you, return to start position, then your left heel. Tap each in front of the other foot.

Side steps Take four steps sideways to one side and four back to the centre.

Hamstring curls With knees slightly bent and feet quite wide apart, kick each foot in turn up towards your buttocks and swing your elbows back.

Side swings Tap your foot to the side, turning your arms to the opposite side with control; don't let your arms pull your body round.

Knee taps Lifting each knee in turn, twist to tap each knee with the opposite hand.

Lunges With knees bent, tap each foot behind you as you swing your arms forwards.

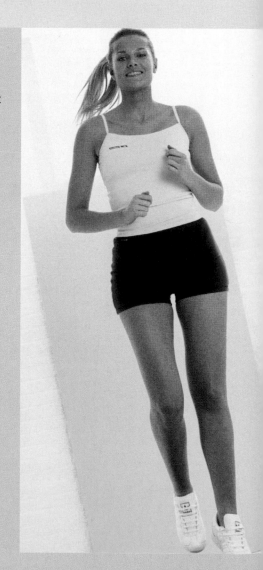

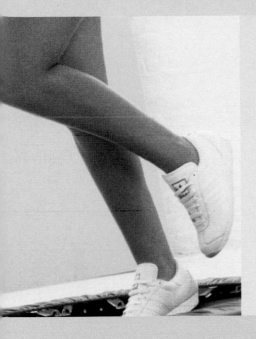

PAIN: NO GAIN

Many people give up on an exercise regime because they started over-enthusiastically and suffered an injury. Instead, start at a level that slightly challenges you and work on up. Move smoothly with control rather than swinging or bouncing. Push your limits gently and take time to perfect each move. Exercises are only effective if carried out correctly. You are wasting your effort as well as risking injury if you do numerous repetitions ('reps') wrongly or force your body past its natural limits. Knees, ankles and lower back are especially vulnerable.

You may ache a little the day after your first few sessions, but you shouldn't feel any pain. If you're exhausted or hobbling, you've been working too hard. Ease off to avoid sabotaging your programme.

To prevent knee injuries, make sure your knees and feet always go in the same direction. Don't change direction at speed.

Above Treat yourself to a good pair of trainers to support and protect your feet while you're exercising. If you have problems, staff in a specialist shop can help you choose the right pair.

Left Maintaining good posture during your workout – spine straight, top of head high – improves efficiency and helps prevent injuries and fatigue.

DOS AND DON'TS
- Don't exercise until three hours after a main meal, or half an hour after a snack or very light breakfast. If you're exercising first thing in the morning, have a drink before you start. (See page 123 for the best time to exercise.)
- Drink water as you need to during the workout.
- Always start with a warm-up (see page 10), and finish with some stretching exercises (see page 11).

Pliés Do some pliés, as in the warm-up (see page 10).

March March on the spot, then take four paces forwards and continue around in a square, and then back.

Repeat the sequence with more energy Raise your knees higher. Lift your heels one at a time and then together during pliés. Kick forwards instead of toe tapping and heel digging. Repeat with strong arm movements. Continue, adding your own dance steps. If you need a break, march on the spot for a while.

arm movements

Add arm movements to increase the exercise intensity.

Pump your fists With your elbows at your side, pump your fists up and down.

Biceps curls Start with your elbows at your sides and your palms facing forwards. Keeping your upper arms still, clench your hands and bring your fists up to your shoulders and back down.

Wave your arms Wave your arms high above your head.

Pec decs Raise your elbows to your sides to shoulder-height, with your fists raised to the ceiling. Bring your elbows towards each other in front of you, then out again.

turn up the heat

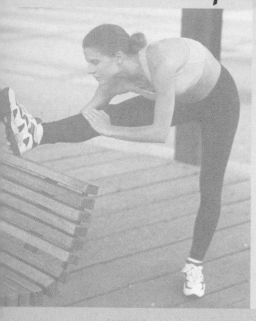

By the end of the first month, if you're exercising regularly, you'll start noticing benefits. The steps that tired you when you started will now seem easy. Add something a bit more demanding – staying careful not to risk an injury that could wreck your shaping-up schedule.

Back up your exercise sessions by becoming more active: walk up escalators, jog to the shops, visit work colleagues instead of emailing them. When you need a break from wedding preparations, take a neighbour's dog for a walk and race it around the park.

running

Jog or run for 4 minutes, sprint for 1 minute and repeat four times. Vary your steps now and then, doing 20 paces with longer strides or lifting your knees high. If you can't keep up the pace, switch to walking briskly until you're ready to jog again. If you're not in a park, watch out for the roads!

skipping

Skip for 1 minute at a comfortable pace, 1 minute at a challenging pace, then 1 minute briskly. Skip fast for 30 seconds, then at a comfortable pace for 30 seconds. Vary the moves by skipping backwards or raising your knees higher. As you progress, skip fast for 45 seconds with only 15 seconds at the easier pace.

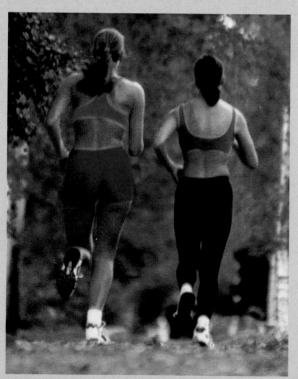

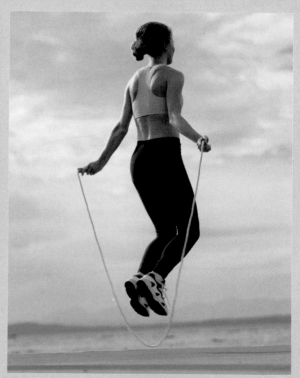

stepping

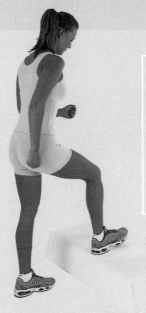

Step up on to the bottom step of your stairs, putting both feet down fully on the step, then step down backwards. Keep stepping up and down for 2 minutes at a comfortable pace. Change your leading foot every so often.

Increase the pace for 2 minutes, then march on the spot for 2 minutes. Do 2 minutes stepping up and down at a comfortable pace, lifting your knees higher. Do 2 minutes at a faster pace, lifting your knees and pumping your arms. Keep your chest lifted throughout and don't turn round. If your knees or back hurt, don't do this exercise.

TOP TIP
Use whatever is available where you happen to be: stairs for a 'step' workout, cans of food to use as hand weights. Models use their ever-changing surroundings to put some variety into their workouts.

ball games

Playing ball games is a sociable way to fit in some aerobic exercise at the weekend. Complete your workout with some muscle toning.

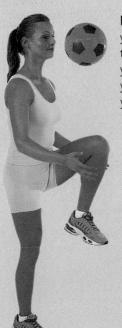

Knee bouncing Bounce a ball off your knees, aiming to keep it off the ground for 100 bounces. Keep your abs pulled in so you can raise your knees high without arching your back.

Ab ball extension Sit with a ball between your heels, and your hands behind to support you. Hold your abs firm to support your back. Lean back and briefly straighten your legs, then return to the starting position. Repeat, sending your feet first to one side, then the other.

STRAIGHT UP
Good form is vital when you're exercising. Poor posture increases your risk of injury and reduces the effectiveness of the exercise – you may even be working the wrong muscles. Try the exercises on page 65 now if bad posture is causing problems.

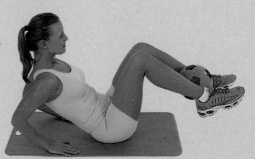

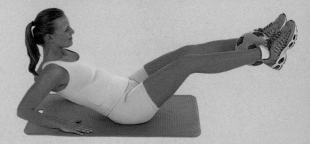

more muscle, less fat

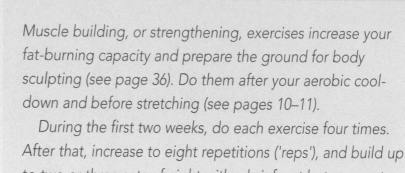

Muscle building, or strengthening, exercises increase your fat-burning capacity and prepare the ground for body sculpting (see page 36). Do them after your aerobic cooldown and before stretching (see pages 10–11).

During the first two weeks, do each exercise four times. After that, increase to eight repetitions ('reps'), and build up to two or three sets of eight with a brief rest between sets.

If you're anxious to start a body sculpting routine early, allow for at least a month of aerobics and muscle building first, then add the body sculpting – don't substitute it.

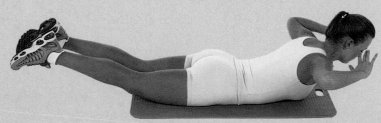

back curls

Lie on your stomach, looking down, and place your hands beside your ears. Squeeze your abs and your buttocks to stop your back arching as you lift your upper body and your legs a short distance off the floor. Hold this position for 5 seconds, then release slowly.

Variation: Superman back curl Extend your arms in front of you. Still looking at the floor, raise your right arm and left leg a little way, and stretch them out like Superman. Return to your start position and repeat on the other side.

squats

Stand with your legs hip-width apart, knees and toes pointing in the same direction. Slowly bend your knees and lower your bottom towards the floor, pushing your bottom out as if about to sit on a chair. Look down and don't let your knees go further forward than your toes. Hold for at least 5 seconds, then slowly return to standing. Try to hold the position longer and go down a little further in the second set of reps.

curl-ups

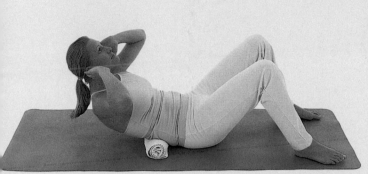

Lie on your back with your knees bent, your feet flat on the floor and your hands on your thighs. If there's enough room to slide a hand beneath the small of your back, let your spine sink closer to the floor, or support your back with a small rolled-up towel.

Slowly lift your head and shoulders, keeping your lower back flat and your head in line with your spine. There should be a tennis ball-sized space between your chin and your chest. Lower slowly to the floor.

Variation: Cup your hands behind your ears, without pushing your head (as shown), to make it harder.

full press-ups

Kneel on all fours with your hands below your shoulders and your fingers pointing forwards. Lift your knees so your body is a straight line from head to heels and all your weight is on your hands and toes. Slowly bend your arms outwards and try to lower your body until your elbows are at right angles. It's better to go down just a short distance than to stick your bottom in the air. Come up slowly and repeat.

If this is too difficult, do the All-Fours Press-Ups instead. If it becomes too easy, go on to Syncopated Press-Ups.

Variation: All-fours press-ups Stay on your hands and knees with your hands a little more than shoulder-width apart, fingers pointing forwards. Lean forward to put some weight on your arms: you won't get any benefit if all your weight is on your knees. Keeping your neck in line with your back, slowly bend your arms outwards and try to touch the floor with your nose.

Variation: Syncopated press-ups Pause when you're halfway down, just above the floor and again halfway up.

MUSCLE-BUILDING TIPS

● Always move slowly.

● Keep breathing steadily, exhaling as you make the effort and inhaling as you return to the starting position.

● Take care not to arch your spine – tightening your abs will help hold your back straight. It's better to do a few reps well than a lot badly.

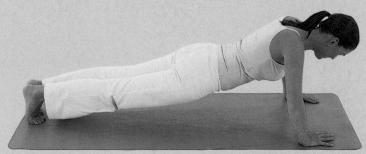

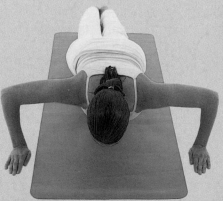

easy everyday toning

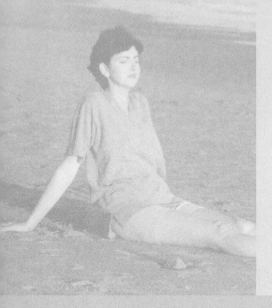

These exercises can be done any time, anywhere, as often as you like during the day. They start gently toning your arms, upper body and waist (focal points in most wedding dresses), while also helping shake off the stiffness that comes from hours of writing wedding invitations!

Shut your eyes for a moment and visualize yourself on a beautiful, peaceful seashore. With waves breaking in a shower of spray, the scene is both relaxing and invigorating. Keeping this feeling in mind, start with some shoulder lifts to help keep your upper body relaxed as you exercise.

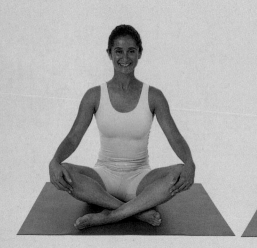

shoulder lifts

Sit or stand with your back straight and your neck long, as though your head is dangling from a string. Lift your shoulders as high as you can. Let your shoulders drop and your arms relax. Feel how low they are and how long your neck is.

Repeat several times. Check every now and then throughout the day to see whether your shoulders have started creeping up. If so, raise and drop them again.

waist stretch

Stand with your feet about hip-width apart. As you breathe in, stretch your arms above your head and interlock your fingers, palms facing upwards.

Leading with your hands, lean slowly to one side as you breathe out – be careful not to tip forwards or backwards. As you breathe in again, return to the centre. Repeat on the other side. Finish by rolling your shoulders forwards and backwards, and shaking any tension out of your arms.

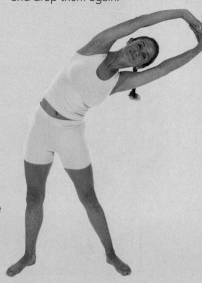

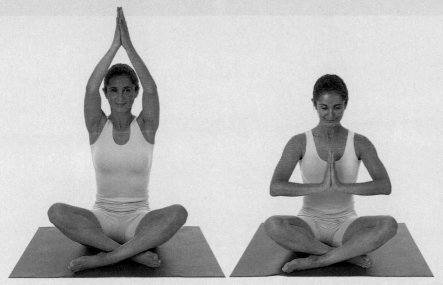

chest toner

Raise your arms above your head and press the palms together in a prayer position. Bring your arms down slowly in front of you with your palms pressed hard together, feeling your chest muscles working. When your forearms are parallel with the floor, let your shoulders relax and then start the exercise from the beginning again.

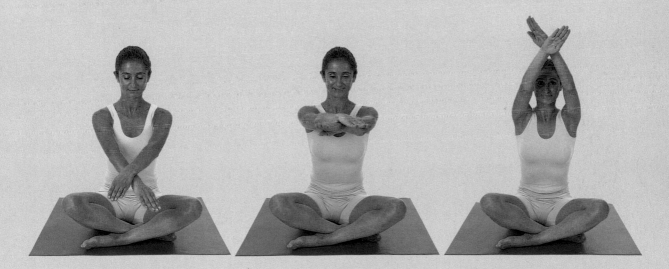

TOP TIP
Speed up your normal walking pace for a simple, everyday, instant workout.

arm crosses

Sit with your arms stretched out in front of you, palms pointing down. Cross them at the wrist, right arm on top. Swing your arms out a few inches apart and bring the left wrist on top. Continue this criss-crossing movement, bringing your arms up as you go, till they're above your head. Keep your shoulders down and your neck long. Criss-cross your arms back down.

eat to lose weight

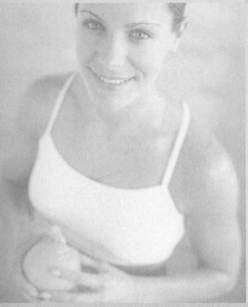

This healthy eating plan will help you shed fat and, importantly, maintain a lower weight. If you suffer from mood swings or fluctuating energy levels, it should even those out, too. Among other things, it takes account of the glycaemic index (GI), which rates foods by the speed at which the body turns them into sugar. High-GI foods raise blood-sugar levels quickly, which can lead to fluctuations. Most of the foods in this plan are low- or medium-GI, which maintain steady levels. This plan should prevent the sudden drop in blood sugar that makes dieters hungry and irritable.

the healthy fat-loss pyramid

This pyramid shows what proportion of different foods to eat each day (the box opposite indicates serving sizes).

White flour, sweet products (such as sugar, cakes, biscuits) and alcohol: not more than one serving, or one unit of alcohol, a day.

Dairy foods (preferably low-fat): one or two servings a day.

Meat, fish, eggs and other high-protein foods: up to two servings a day. Include oily fish at least twice a week.

Nuts, seeds, legumes and their oils: one to three servings a day. One of these can be replaced with butter.

Starchy foods (i.e. wholemeal bread, wholegrain cereals, non-instant rice, pasta): two to four servings a day.

Fruit: three or four servings a day, not more than one from dried fruit. Fresh is best, otherwise canned in juice.

Vegetables: unlimited amounts, at least five servings a day.

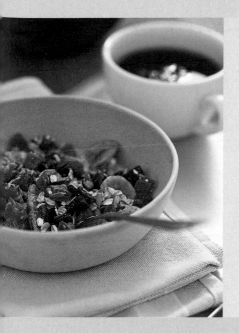

do you need to lose weight?

Your body mass index (BMI) is a rough estimate of whether you are overweight. It's harder to lose weight if you're already a healthy BMI, as your body is trying to stay healthy.

To find your BMI, divide your weight in kilos (kg) by the square of your height in metres (m). So, if you're 1.65 m tall and weigh 57 kg, your BMI is 57 divided by (1.65 x 1.65 =) 2.72, which comes to just under 21. Alternatively, multiply your weight in pounds by 700 and divide it by the square of your height in inches. So, if you're 5 ft 5 in tall and weigh 9 stone, or 126 pounds, that's (126 x 700 =) 88,200, divided by (65 x 65 =) 4,225: just under 21.

A BMI under 19 is considered to be underweight, over 25 is overweight and over 30 is obese. Between 19 and 25 is healthy.

Above Don't miss out on eating breakfast, every day: skipping breakfast has been linked with weight gain, as it increases sugar cravings. A bowl of wholegrain cereal and dried fruit makes a healthy snack, too.

READY RECKONER

One serving is 75 g (3 oz). For most foods, that's roughly as much as you can hold in your hand. To get a feeling for portion size, weigh all your food for the first week.

- Meat and fish: a piece as big and thick as the palm of your hand
- Bread rolls: the size of your fist
- Bread: one slice
- Cheese: a 2.5-cm (1-in) cube, about the size of the top joint of your thumb
- Pasta: a bundle of dry spaghetti, 2.5 cm (1 in) across, or two fistfuls of cooked pasta
- Pasta sauce: a ladleful as big as your fist
- Fruit juice: a 150 ml (1/4 pint) glass
- Berry-sized fruit: a small bowl of strawberries, grapes, etc.
- Small fruit: two plums, satsumas, etc.
- Medium-sized fruit: one apple, pear, etc.
- Large fruit: one big slice of melon, etc.
- Cooked fruit and vegetables: two to three tablespoonfuls
- Beans and pulses: two tablespoonfuls
- Salad: a small mixed side salad
- Dried fruit, nuts and seeds: about a handful
- Oils and fats: a teaspoonful

beauty diet

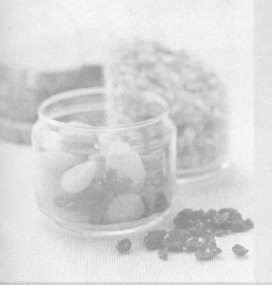

This eating plan will keep your weight down, improve your health and increase your vitality. But above all, it's a beauty diet. A high-protein low-carb diet can cause a dull complexion and killer breath. An ultra low-fat diet is likely to cause premature wrinkling, while a crash diet will leave you looking haggard. A low-sugar diet, rich in vegetables and omega-3 oils, however, will give your skin a peachy glow.

'Junk food' is usually laden with unhealthy fats, while foods labelled 'low-fat' tend to contain more sugar and/or artificial sweeteners. All of these make skin look old and dull.

breakfast

Never skip this vital meal: if you're in a hurry, take some fruit with you. (Don't buy 'breakfast bars', which tend to be high in fat and sugar.) Make a low-GI choice for long-lasting energy, such as:
- Porridge with low-fat milk and a sprinkling of raisins
- Low-fat yogurt with fruit
- Muesli or low-sugar cereals with chopped apple and strawberries and low-fat milk (flaked cereals have a higher GI, while toasted cereals are laden with fat)
- Granary or barley toast with yeast extract and a fruit juice

lunch

Choose a high-protein option to keep you alert in the afternoon, such as:
- Tuna sandwich with mustard-and-cress and an apple
- Bean or hard-boiled egg salad with lots of green leaves
- Organic chicken with steamed vegetables
- Spanish-style omelette with plenty of diced vegetables

dinner

Go for a high-carbohydrate meal to help you relax, such as:
- Pasta with tomato sauce
- Vegetable curry with rice
- Beans on toast
- Baked potato with cottage cheese and salad

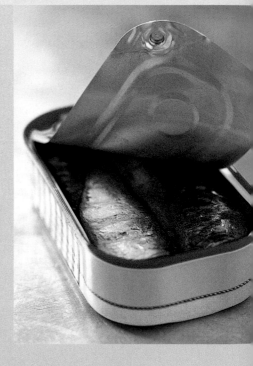

Above When wedding planning tasks pile up or guests drop out, eat more oily fish – the omega-3 oils from fatty fish have been found to lift low moods. Longer term, the effects on your skin will cheer you up, too.

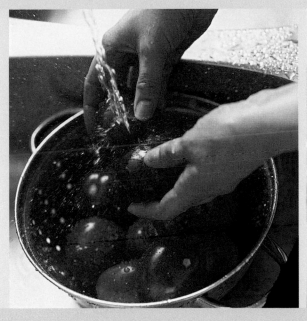

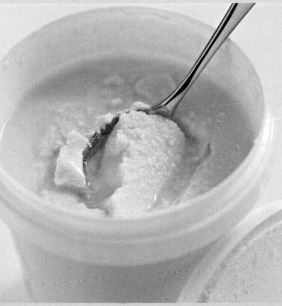

Above right Eat organic foods when possible, especially meat and dairy produce such as yogurt, since these otherwise come from industrially raised animals dosed with drugs and chemicals.

Above You don't buy the cheapest shoes you can find, so why skimp on food, which has more effect on your looks? Buy the best you can afford: fresh, natural and unprocessed.

snacks

Have two snacks a day to fill any gaps, such as:
- A handful of nuts and raisins
- A serving of fruit
- A rye crispbread with cheese
- Oatcakes spread with mashed banana – a relaxing bedtime snack

evening

If you're an evening nibbler, save at least one snack to have then. Otherwise, don't eat after 9pm – that's when you're likely to munch automatically and finish the whole pack.

oil reserves

We all need some oil, or fat, in our diet to lubricate our skin from the inside (as well as to stay alive). The most effective are those containing omega-3 fats, and the best source of these is oily fish.
- Eat oily fish at least twice a week: mackerel, wild salmon, tuna, trout, herrings, sardines or bass.
- Linseed (flaxseed) oil has many of the same benefits. Use it in salad dressings, since it doesn't heat well.
- Olive oil is good for cooking or salads.
- Evening primrose oil, as a food supplement, has an almost miraculously beautifying effect on hair, nails and skin. But check with your doctor before taking any supplement, and don't overdose.

IN A NUTSHELL...

Eat more
- Omega-3 oils
- Vegetables

Eat less
- Sugar
- Processed food

---

low-cal variety

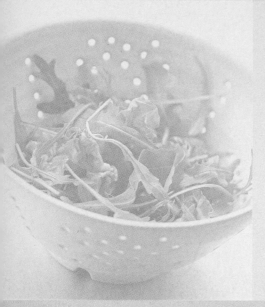

Processed foods are made from a very small number of basic ingredients: the long lists on their labels are mainly additives. Vegetables and fruit in literally thousands of varieties give you a far more interesting, varied diet. Trawl market stalls, explore greengrocers' shops, search through delicatessens. Find what your supermarket has to offer, in the ethnic and specialist sections as well as the freezers and fresh produce shelves. Rinse everything well before you cook or eat it. Buy organic when possible, especially salads, leafy vegetables and anything bought out of season.

slimming with vegetables

Most vegetables contain very few calories and plenty of healthy fibre, which fills you up and helps you digest your food. They're also low in fat. Deep-fried and roast veg gain most of their high calorie count from the fat they're cooked in, so save these for occasional treats.

To lose weight, try eating slightly smaller portions, and don't have more than one serving a day of root vegetables such as potatoes and parsnips, which are high on the GI scale. But if you're hungry or you get the munchies, always fill up on vegetables.

Scientists have found that extra vegetables and fruit are more effective than fatty foods in filling you up, resulting in a lighter but more satisfying meal. In addition, they provide too many health benefits to list: no other food group comes near.

get experimental

Instead of processed food flavourings cooked up in a lab, discover your own favourite tastes.

Experiment with adding different herbs and spices while you're preparing food. Add them to stir-fries, sprinkle them over grilled vegetables, mix them into salad dressings, include some extra in cooked dishes.

Herbs can be bought dried or fresh in pots to grow on your windowsill. Follow your nose to ethnic shops with mounds of fresh produce on display, including herbs and spices from afar – then check what they are and how to use them.

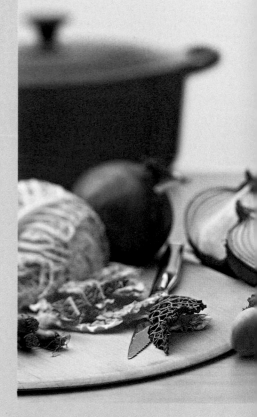

Above One of the easiest meals you can make in advance is a casserole: your choice of meat, vegetables and herbs, chopped up and cooking in the oven while you get on with something else.

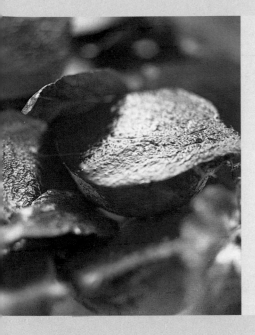

GREAT WAYS WITH VEGETABLES
- Stir-fry vegetables with one or two teaspoons of olive oil. Add garlic, ginger, herbs or a dash of soy sauce to taste.
- Steam them over broth or boiling water flavoured with herbs.
- Boil them up for soup – leftovers are fine in this.
- Chop them raw into salads.
- Grate them into sandwiches.
- Grill them or cook them in the oven, brushed with oil, to release all the sweetness.
- Add more vegetables to ready-made sauces for pasta or meat.
- Cook some frozen vegetables and add to a can or carton of soup.
- For extra flavour when cooking vegetables, add garlic or your choice of herbs, or a little organic bacon.

Above Cooked beetroot is popular in salads, but why not try it in soups and stews, too? It's as delicious hot as cold, and forms the basis of some classic dishes such as the eastern European soup, bortsch.

salads can be interesting

Bored with lettuce and tomatoes? Try alternatives such as alfalfa and other sprouts, asparagus, beetroot, celery, chicory, watercress, baby dandelion leaves, endive, fennel, artichokes, radishes, mushrooms, edible seaweed and baby spinach. Some of these need to be cooked, so check before biting them! Decorate them with edible flowers, such as marigold or nasturtium.

Adding raw or cold cooked vegetables makes a salad more filling. Green ones work especially well: try peas, mangetouts, sugar snap peas or runner beans.

The basic vinaigrette dressing consists of extra virgin olive oil, vinegar and a pinch of salt. Explore your local delicatessen for numerous different vinegars, oils and mustards to vary the taste of your salads. The lightest dressing is just a dash of vinegar, or a squirt of lemon or lime juice, with whatever dried herbs you like.

fruit

Fruit (particularly dried fruit) is higher in sugar than vegetables, so eat just two to three servings a day if you want to lose weight. Fresh is best, otherwise canned in juice, not syrup.

Fruit with a low GI (see page 20) include apples, berries, cherries, citrus fruit, white grapes, kiwi fruit, peaches, pears, plums and strawberries.

Once your weight has stabilized, fruit joins vegetables as the basis for your healthy diet, and you can eat as much of it as you like.

WHY EAT VEGETABLES?
Most vegetables are low in calories. Packed with nutrition, they can be eaten in almost unlimited quantities, even on a weight-loss diet. Fresh or frozen are best. Bottled or canned are fine, but watch out for fatty sauces. Try to eat every colour: green, greenish-white (such as onions), yellow, red, purple and orange.

planning for beauty

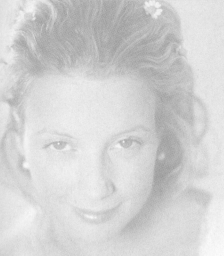

Starting six months in advance gives you plenty of time to create a beauty regime that works for you, and build it into your everyday routine. You've left yourself enough leeway to try a few different options, discard any that don't suit you and fine-tune those you find most beneficial. The results of some will soon be noticeable, motivating you to continue. If you get into the habit of sleeping eight hours a night, for example, you'll soon see an improvement in the skin around your eyes. This unhurried approach also allows you to make long-term changes that will deliver their benefits in time.

things to think about

No make-up can create the glow of an unblemished, even-textured complexion. So begin by tackling any existing beauty problems.

● Make an appointment with a dermatologist if you have any skin problems such as acne that need to be treated. Any serious cosmetic treatments you're planning, such as a chemical peel, should be done now to allow time for healing.

● If you want a tattoo removed, check there will be time for the scar to heal completely before the wedding; otherwise, you'll be safer using camouflage make-up.

● Facials can work wonders, and they show their best effects after regular treatments. Either book a series of monthly professional facials or start doing it yourself (see page 28). Start exfoliating regularly, too.

● If you're wearing a backless or low-cut dress, you could also consider treatments for those areas, to brighten skin that is usually hidden. If you're doing it yourself, simply continue your facial routine down to your chest and back.

make-up

Now is the time to make an appointment with a make-up artist, either to discuss having it done professionally or, if you're doing it yourself on the day, to learn how to do your own make-up. Beauty counters at department stores will often give lessons, too.

If you're thinking of using fake tan, try it out now: remember to exfoliate first for an even finish. If you get any fake tan in the wrong

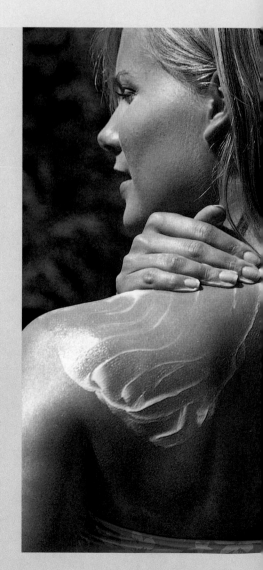

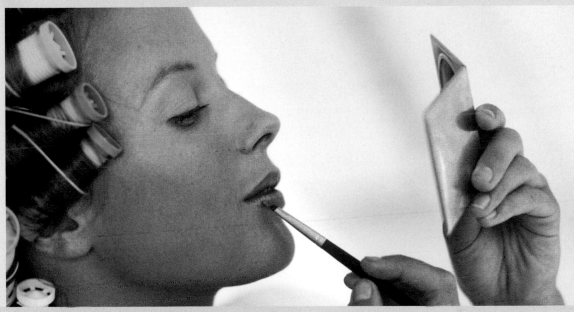

Above Make-up for a wedding is very different from your everyday routine, especially if you don't often wear white. Even if you or a friend will be doing it on the day, treat yourself to one professional lesson, then practise at home.

Left If your dress will reveal your back or shoulders, remember to give these areas the same kind of care you give your face. Start nourishing and exfoliating now.

place, rub it with whitening toothpaste, leave for a few minutes and it should rub off. This is also a good time to start trying any other creams or cosmetics you'd like to use, bearing in mind that you don't want to try anything new in the final few weeks in case of adverse reactions.

top form

It can be helpful to wear a top with a similar neckline to your wedding dress when choosing your hairstyle, make-up, head-dress and bouquet. Wearing a colour close to that of your dress will also help you see at a glance whether something will work or not. A make-up palette applied against a dark top may look very different against a pale dress.

Take a friend along to appointments for moral support and an honest opinion. But also carry a digital or Polaroid camera around so you can take time afterwards to decide what you like best. Have pictures taken from the side and back as well as in front.

smoking wrinkles

If you smoke, give up now. By robbing your body of oxygen, smoking dulls your skin, causes premature wrinkling and reduces your ability to exercise. Giving up is not as difficult as it may seem. The physical withdrawal symptoms are over in a few days; after that, it's just habit. But if you don't, deep down, want to give up – perhaps because you fear you'll put on weight or you enjoy sharing it with friends – the psychological cravings can be strong. If you don't give up now, it's probably best to wait until after the wedding.

TOP TIP
Moisturize your neck whenever you moisturize your face – take the cream around under your ears and down into your cleavage. If you have dry skin, leave a moisturizing mask on overnight once a week.

a prettier face

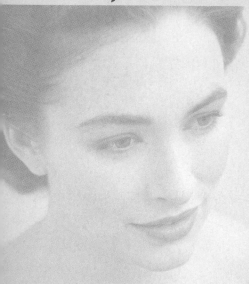

Once a week, set aside time for a facial and carry out the whole of the regime below to improve the look of your skin and hair. Try to make this part of an unhurried evening ritual, which you end with a warm bath and an early night.

On the other nights of the week, do a shorter routine (see Daily Facial Routine opposite), using your normal moisturizer instead of the essential oil at the massage stage. If you have oily skin, you may not wish to moisturize every day – in any case, do treat yourself to the weekly massage, using a light moisturizer instead of essential oils.

shinier hair

Shampoo your hair and towel dry. Apply an intensive conditioning treatment or mix up your own with half a cup of warm (not hot) almond oil and ten drops of lavender essential oil. Apply this to your hair using gentle massage movements to stimulate the scalp, then tie a plastic carrier bag around your hair to increase the rate at which the treatment penetrates the hair. Leave this on while you carry out your facial. After the moisturizing and massaging, shampoo your hair again, rinse well and towel dry.

younger face

This exercise tones facial muscles and reduces the muscle tension that can hinder circulation.

Sit comfortably, resting your palms on your legs. Inhale, then exhale slowly; while you do this, open your eyes and mouth as wide as possible. Very slowly, stick your tongue out and down as far as it will go (without straining), and you'll feel the muscles around your face tighten. Now stiffen your arms and fingers. Hold this 'Lion' position for as long as you can, then slowly relax.

beautifully clean

Cleanse the skin with your normal cleanser, or mix up a natural cleanser using a tablespoon of natural yogurt and a teaspoon of lemon juice. Dab this off the skin with a tissue, then rinse with cool water.

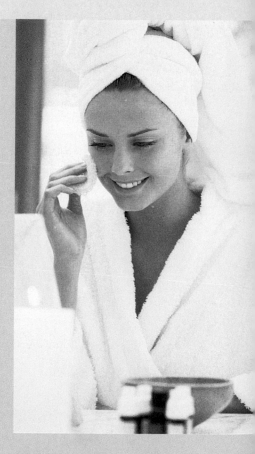

Above Thoroughly cleansing and wiping off all traces of cleanser is especially important before steaming, to stop dirt being pulled deeper into your skin. Wipe gently without dragging the skin.

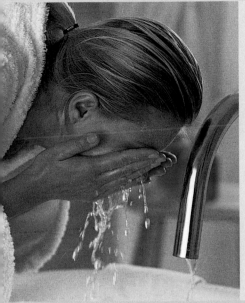

skin polish

Use a gentle store-bought exfoliator or add enough water to a teaspoon of sugar to mix to a smooth paste – make sure that it isn't too thick and scratchy or too liquid. Rinse off thoroughly.

steam clean

Steaming helps release any toxins and impurities that may be just under the skin's surface, blocking circulation. Hold your face about 10 cm (4 in) above a bowl of hot (not boiling) water for 2–3 minutes. Intensify the effects of the steam by placing a towel over your head to trap the vapours, but don't do this if you have asthma because it can irritate the respiratory tract.

Above Splash your face with cool water to tighten pores and make your skin glow. If your eyes are tired after poring over menus or writing lists, soothe them with a splash of cold water on your closed eyelids.

splash and firm

Cold water is a great skin tightener. Simply splash the skin 20–30 times quickly with cool or cold water, then pat dry with a towel. Don't use very cold water on steam nights, because the dramatic change in temperature can overstress the skin and lead to broken veins.

moisturize and massage

Add two drops of your chosen oil (use camomile for dry skins, rose for oily skins and carrot seed for mature skins) to a carrier oil like grapeseed. If you're pregnant, use just the grapeseed oil. Now apply the oil, massaging the skin as you go.

1 **Work upwards** Start at your chin, gently smoothing the skin upwards with the pads of your fingers; don't tug the skin, just smooth it. Now drum your fingers lightly, moving up the jawline. Repeat five times.
2 **Cheeky moves** Repeat these moves over your cheeks. Now quickly pat the cheeks and jaw five to ten times; start lightly but then get firmer.
3 **Roll it out** Stroke up around the temples and up the forehead. Repeat the drumming motion. When you get to the middle of the forehead, use the index fingers of each hand alternately to brush rapidly upwards from the middle of your brows to the hairline; this should feel like a smooth, rolling movement.
4 **Finishing touches** Lastly, treat the under-eye area. Dab a little oil along the socket bone below each eye (oils should never go directly on the eye area), and massage this in well, using gentle upward strokes. Finish by lightly drumming your fingers along each socket bone.

DAILY FACIAL ROUTINE
Do the whole of the above regime once a week. Do a shorter routine on a daily basis:

- Younger face
- Beautifully clean
- Splash and firm
- Moisturize and massage

a flattering dress

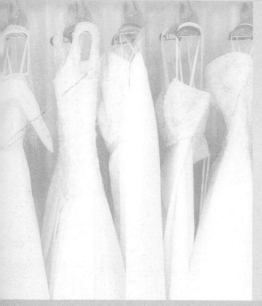

It's the biggest dressing-up day in most of our lives. And there's a bewildering choice of styles, from Cinderella ballgowns to designs hot from the catwalks. So take your time and enjoy choosing.

It's likely to work best if you choose something that suits you as you are now, rather than the fantasy bride you may have carried in your head since you were 12. On the other hand, very modern styles soon look dated in photos. If this would disappoint you rather than bring a nostalgic smile to your face, consider something classic.

dress sense

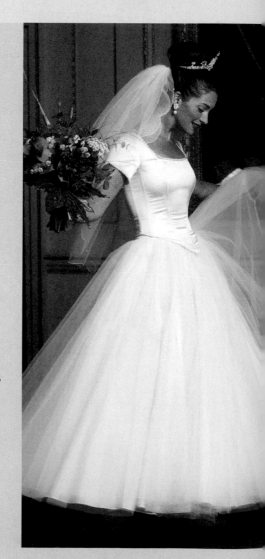

Factors to weigh up include the changeable, such as your weight and hair; unchangeable, such as your build and height; personal – your favourite style and wedding theme; and practical, such as cost, and whether you want to have your bridesmaids matching. With these in mind, consider your best options.

The traditional ballgown has a fitted bodice and full skirt. Hips and thighs vanish under its generous folds and, although the bodice looks terrific on a tiny waist, it's surprisingly forgiving to less honed figures. The fullness of the skirt will balance a low, off-the-shoulder neckline, showing off a bigger bride's bosom and making the most of a smaller one. Petticoats and a bustle can be added to puff the skirt out even more, though these are best avoided by brides who are tiny or very tall.

The A-line, or princess, style has vertical seams falling from the shoulders or the waist to create a flared skirt. Graceful and easy to wear, it skims over imperfections and makes almost anyone look taller and slimmer. Yet tall, slim brides can wear it, too.

Most brides opt for an A-line or a ballgown, so you'll find the greatest range of choices in these. The other styles are harder to wear, though they look stunning if you have the shape to carry them off.

An empire-line dress fits snugly over the bust and falls straight, or with very little flare, from a high waist. Not for the plump, this is flattering to a small bust or a straight-up-and-down shape.

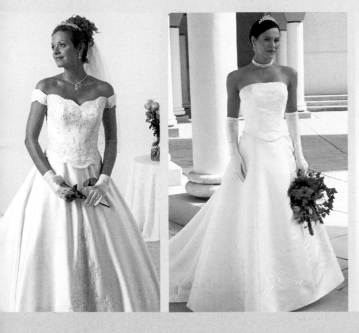

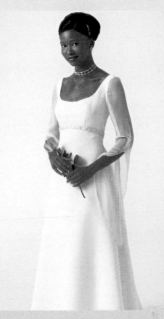

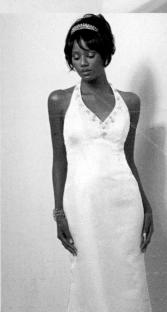

Above left to right The classic dress styles: ballgown, A-line, empire-line and sheath.

Left Not for fairy-tale princesses only, a full-skirted ballgown hides a multitude of sins. A fitted bodice with a point at the waist persuades your torso into the perfect shape.

A sheath, fitted all the way down, shows off a body that's flawlessly slim but not too skinny.

A mermaid, or fit-and-release, style is tightly fitted down to the thighs and then flares out. Difficult for most women; stupendous if you are slender but shapely.

Then there's the choice of sleeveless, strapless, low-cut or high-necked. Draping and details add shape to a flat chest. You can minimize a large bust with a simple bodice, or celebrate it with a strapless style – as long as the tight bodice doesn't cause bulges. If you plan to wear heirloom jewellery, or have a strong preference for a particular head-dress or hairstyle, these will influence your choice of neckline. Take your time, a digital or Polaroid camera and friends who will give their honest opinion. But in the end, remember it's your choice.

beauty goals

Your choice of dress will set specific goals, depending on what parts of your body are revealed or emphasized. But don't choose something that's far too small, or that depends on a total body transformation. Putting pressure on yourself rarely works – you'll just add masses of stress at this busy time.

Choose a dress that makes you look your best now, in a style and fabric that won't be ruined if it has to be altered. Book the dressmaker, and check how much time will be needed for alterations. Remember that toned muscles look shapelier, but may take up more space.

LOOK AT ME NOW
It's probably the most expensive garment you'll ever buy, and you'll only wear it once. If you don't want to keep it as an heirloom, consider hiring the dress. For less than the cost of a cheap purchase, you could wear a designer gem that will shine forever in your photos. Just make sure you can change the size if necessary.

hair affairs

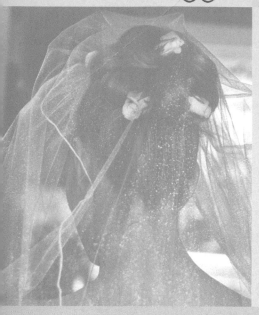

Planning a change of hairstyle for your wedding? Now is the time to try out anything radical such as a perm or a new colour. You may love it, hate it or want to adapt a few details. Either way, you've got time to try new ideas.

Start bringing your hair into peak condition. If it is already in good shape, there's no need to make changes unless you feel like trying something new. Strong treatments can damage hair, if they aren't necessary.

On sunny days, instead of sunscreen, protect both your hair and your complexion by wearing a wide-brimmed hat.

hair help

If your hair needs some help, this is the time to break any habits that have damaged it and create a beauty regime that suits both you and your hair.

Don't...
- Brush hair when it's wet.
- Use hot tools on hair, or dry it with excessive heat.
- Pull it back too tightly.

Do...
- Try protective or restorative treatments to discover which ones suit you. As with skin care, one woman's moisturizing treatment is another's oil slick.
- Try an occasional deep-conditioning treatment if your hair is dry, or see whether your hair responds to washing more or less often. If it's oily, try applying conditioner to the ends only.
- Use protective treatments when you go swimming and, if you're blonde, stay out of heavily chlorinated swimming pools, which can cause discoloration.

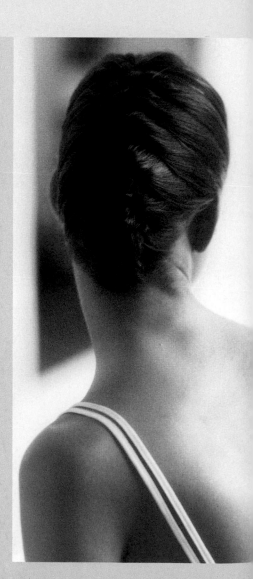

a new style

If you're bored with your hair, or if you've never really found a style you like, what better time to sort it out? Ask friends for recommendations and try out different hairdressers till you find a style you love.

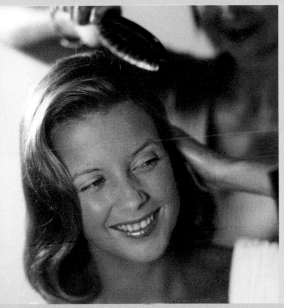

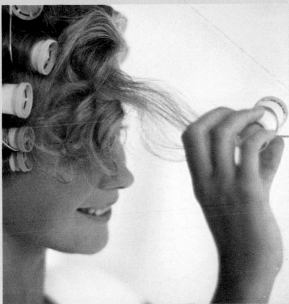

Above If you or a friend will be doing your hair on the day, book a session for both of you with your hairdresser, to decide on the style and make sure you have the technique. Then practise at home.

Left Putting your hair up in a sleek, unfussy style gives the impression of a long, elegant neck. It also creates the perfect background for an ornate head-dress or a full veil.

If you want your hair done professionally on the day, it's not too early to find out whether your regular hairdresser can do your wedding hair, or whether they can recommend a wedding specialist. Consider paying the extra for the stylist to come to you at the house – coming back from the salon on your wedding day in wind or rain could add stress and undo all their efforts.

If you or a friend will be doing your hair, organize an appointment at which the stylist will teach you both how to create the style you want on the day. Then practise at home.

hairstyle, dress style

Long, loose hair looks fresh and lovely with a simple dress style. You want the look to be flowing, not straggling, so sacrifice the last few inches if it's thin at the ends. Make sure it's in top condition and doesn't clash with any detailing at the neckline. Hair grows at the rate of about 1 cm (^{1}/2 in) a month. If you're starting to grow it now, allow time for trims to keep it in perfect shape.

A formal dress generally calls out for an **up or half-up style**. Upswept looks best with a high neckline, and gives the impression of an elegantly long neck. Leave at least some tendrils loose if your dress is low cut. While you're trying out different hairstyles, put on any jewellery that you plan to wear on the day.

Think about your **head-dress**, too. Is there a style you'd love, and will you need to arrange your hair to suit it? Or will you choose the head-dress to suit the way you want to wear your hair? Will you be wearing a **veil,** and if so, how will that affect your hair?

HEAD OFF TROUBLE
Hair can be badly affected by poor diet, stress and hormonal upheaval, any of which may overtake you when you're organizing a major change in your life. If you notice this, it's a useful warning: remember that you're planning a joyful event, not trying to make yourself ill.

body sculpting

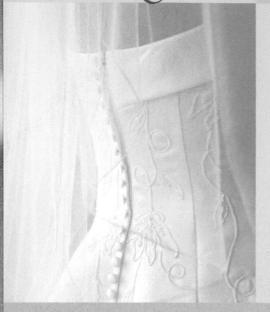

The aerobic and muscle-building work you've been doing has been preparing your body for a more focused sculpting programme. From now on, you'll be targeting the areas your wedding dress will show off. Toning the right muscles can change your shape and improve the appearance of your skin.

First, try on your dress to help you decide what part of your body needs the most work. Are flabby upper arms visible when you wave? Does your back, in a low-cut bodice, look bony or too soft? Does the clingy fabric you love accentuate your stomach or bottom?

body-sculpting basics

To see the most benefit, you'll need to work on a specific area of your body every other day. You can do all three body-sculpting workouts (see pages 38–43) once or twice a week if you have the time. For a more demanding workout, use heavier handweights, going up one level at a time. If this is too heavy, do more reps instead.

Carry on with your aerobics You should still be doing aerobic exercise for at least half an hour, two or three times a week. If you're intending to lose more weight, do 30 minutes to an hour of aerobic work every other day, followed by a few minutes of muscle building and then a body-sculpting session. As always, stop if anything hurts.

Warm up before body sculpting Start with a warm-up (see page 10), then do a specific warm-up for the area you're tackling (see opposite). Repeat each movement eight to ten times. When you go straight from aerobic exercise to body sculpting, don't do a warm-up in between.

> **BREATH AND MUSCLE CONTROL**
> Good posture makes the exercises more effective and protects you from injury. So keep your spine straight – not arched – and tighten your abdominal muscles ('abs') as you do each exercise. It should feel as though the muscles below the waist are lifting upwards and your navel is pushing towards your spine.
>
> Practise breathing fully without loosening your abs. Breathe steadily, exhaling with the effort, and don't hold your breath.

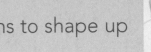

upper-body warm-up

Stand tall with your abs pulled in. Place your hands on your shoulders and try to draw full circles with your elbows, forwards and then backwards.

Body curls Stretch your arms up to the ceiling, leaning slightly backwards. Then stretch them out to the sides at shoulder level and bend your knees. Curl your body forwards and let your head and arms hang down. Then curl upwards to a standing position.

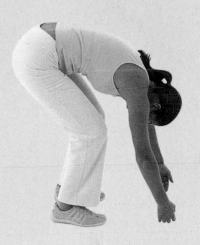

stomach and waist warm-up

Stand tall with your feet hip-width apart and your hands on your hips. Circle your hips as widely as possible several times in each direction, keeping your upper body fairly straight. Then make circles with your upper body, keeping your hips still. Then lean to each side in turn, facing forwards and letting your hands slide down and up your thighs.

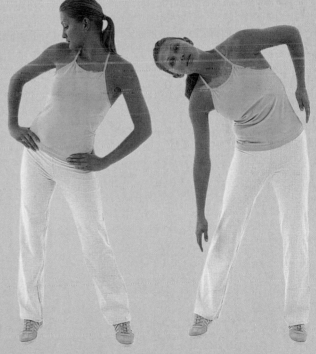

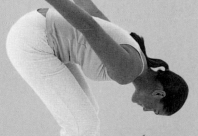

bottom and hips warm-up

Stand tall with your arms stretched above your head, your abs and thigh muscles held tight. Bend your knees, lean forwards energetically and swing your arms till they're up behind your back and your head is hanging down. Return to the start position.

shapelier arms and chest

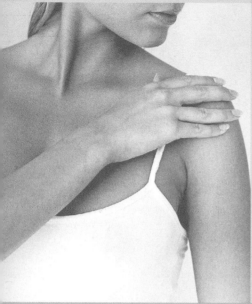

If you'll be wearing a sleeveless or low-cut dress, you'll almost definitely benefit from an upper-body workout. Do these exercises, plus the Superman Back Curl and Press-Ups from pages 16–17, every other day. Start with a warm-up and end with the arm stretches on page 11.

When working one arm at a time, do a full set before swapping to the other side. Do eight repetitions of each exercise, or on each side, for the first two weeks. After that, work up gradually to two or three sets of 12. Use heavier weights if this becomes easy. Move slowly and with control.

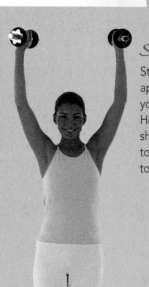

shoulder press

Stand with your feet hip-width apart, knees slightly bent, and your palms facing each other. Hold a weight in each hand at shoulder-height, then raise towards the ceiling and lower to shoulder-level.

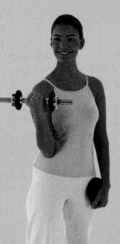

seated row

Sit on a chair and lean forward to rest your torso on your lap. Let your head hang down over your knees and your arms hang by your sides, palms facing each other. Holding weights, lift your outstretched arms to shoulder-height, then lower to the floor.

biceps curls

Stand with your feet hip-width apart, knees slightly bent, and your palms facing forwards. Holding a weight in your right hand, raise it to shoulder-height and back down, keeping your elbow close to your side.

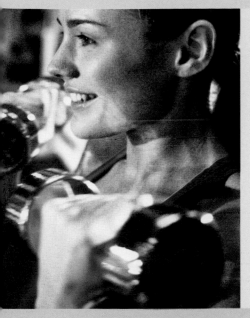

USING WEIGHTS

All these exercises can be done without weights, or holding a can of beans, but you'll gain most benefit in the least time with a set of hand weights, about 1–4 kg (2–8 lb).

To choose the right weight, hold one while you do ten repetitions of an exercise. The tenth rep should be difficult. If you're struggling before you reach ten, use a lighter weight until you build up strength. Try before you buy, with ten biceps curls and ten triceps extensions. The one that's right for biceps curls is the heaviest you'll need to start with. Triceps extensions are more strenuous, so the weight that challenges you on the tenth rep is the lightest you'll need.

It's more important than ever to keep your abs engaged, back straight and shoulders down when you're using weights.

triceps extension

Stand with your feet hip-width apart, knees slightly bent, and your palms facing each other. Holding a weight in your left hand, raise your arm above your head and support the elbow with your right hand. Bend your elbow to lower the weight behind your shoulder, then straighten it again.

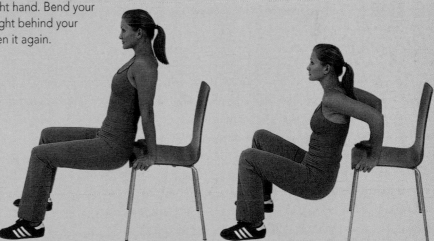

triceps dip

This upper-arm firmer uses body weight instead of hand weights. Sit on the edge of a chair that won't tip up, with your feet flat on the floor, knees at right angles and your hands gripping the edge beside you. Move forwards off the edge of the chair, so you're supported by your arms, being careful not to lock your elbows. Lower your bottom towards the floor until your elbows are bent at right angles, then come back up till they're straight again.

a trimmer waist and stomach

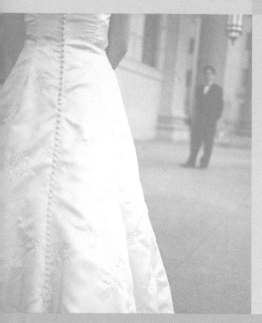

If you're planning to wear a traditional ballgown, hone your waist to emphasize the sumptuous curves of your skirt and neckline. This creates the illusion of a perfect hourglass shape, regardless of your actual bust or hip size. If you're wearing a clingy fabric or a fitted dress, a sleek silhouette will make you glad you worked on your abdominals – no one remembers to hold their tummy in all day! Even if your dress doesn't accentuate your waist, strong abs will support your back, helping you stay poised throughout the day. Do these exercises, plus the Curl-Ups (see page 17), every other day.

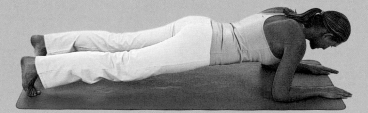

tension hold

Get down on all fours, resting on your knees and elbows, keeping your back straight. Extend one leg behind you and press your toes into the floor, then do the same with the other foot. You are now supported on your elbows and toes. Tighten your abdominal muscles to keep your body as straight as a plank, without sagging or lifting your bottom up. Hold for 15 seconds. As you get stronger, hold for up to 30 seconds and repeat up to four times.

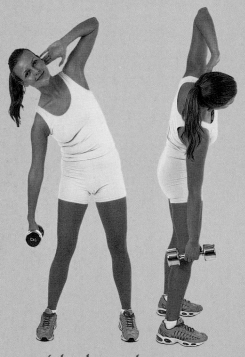

side bends

Stand with your feet hip-width apart, your right arm, holding a weight, by your side with the palm facing inwards and your left hand cupping the back of your head. Holding your abs in firmly, slide your right hand as far as possible down your thigh and your left elbow towards the ceiling, taking 10 seconds to go down and return. Move as if sandwiched front and back between two panes of glass, without leaning forwards or backwards. Do a whole set before repeating on the other side.

TOP TIP
A rubber resistance band makes a compact and portable substitute for hand weights.

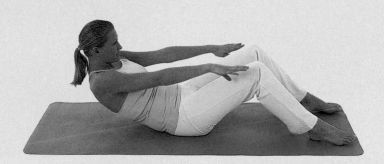

roll-down

Sit on the floor with your knees bent, feet flat on the floor and your arms straight out in front of you. Slowly lean back and lower yourself towards the floor, thinking about pressing the vertebrae towards the floor one by one. Stop halfway down – or before that if you start to collapse – and hold the position for 10 seconds before coming slowly back up. Build up to five repetitions, with brief rests in between.

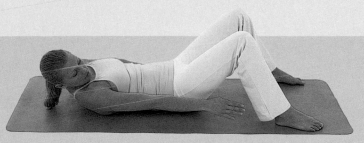

side pulses

Lie on your back with your knees bent, feet pressed firmly into the floor and your arms by your sides. Curl your head and shoulders up off the floor, leaving space between your chin and your chest. Tilt your body to the right and reach towards your right shin with your right hand. Perform 20 small pulsing movements towards the shin, feeling your oblique muscles contract, then release back to the starting position. Repeat on the left side. Build up to five sets on each side, with brief rests in between.

stretches

Finish by lying on your back, hugging your knees into your chest to stretch out your lower back. Rock from side to side to release any tension in the back. Put your feet on the floor with your knees bent and gently drop your knees first to one side, then the other. Then stretch your arms and legs out along the floor and make yourself as long as possible. Hold each stretch for at least 30 seconds, then let your muscles relax as you lie on the floor.

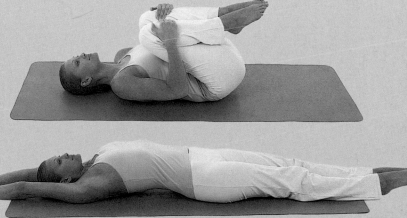

41

sleek hips and thighs

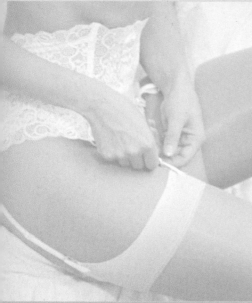

This is the one big event in which even the most body-conscious woman probably needn't worry too much about the shape of her hips and thighs, since many of the most popular styles of wedding dress emphasize the upper body. A less conventional choice, however, may draw the eye to other parts. You may have chosen a short skirt, or a slit up the side or a slender sheath that offers nowhere to hide. A targeted workout can ensure you're looking your best on the big day. And, of course, some work on your hips and thighs will pay off when you head for the beach on your honeymoon.

hip and thigh sculpting

- **Start** by doing eight repetitions of each exercise below (eight on each side, where appropriate) in the first two weeks, plus the Squats from page 16 and the Pliés from page 10.
- **Build up** to two or three sets of eight to 12. Be careful to hold in your abs throughout and not to arch or slump your back.
- **Finish** with the leg stretches from page 11, and the Seated Twist Stretch opposite.

TOP TIP
Never eat more food at a meal than you could hold in your two cupped hands.

bottom pulse

Lie on your back with your knees bent and feet on the floor. Lift your hips off the floor as high as you can without hurting your back. Using your buttock muscles, raise and lower your hips in eight small pulsing movements up and down. After a brief pause, do another eight and then another eight: this counts as one set.

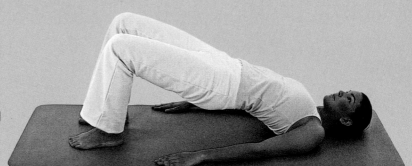

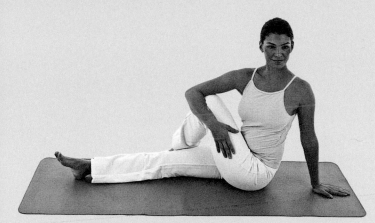

seated twist stretch

Sit on the floor with your legs outstretched in front of you. Bend your left leg, cross it over the right leg and place the left foot flat on the floor. Turn your torso towards the left and wrap your right arm around the left knee. Pull the knee into your body so you can feel a stretch in the left buttock. Hold for 10–15 seconds, then release. Repeat on the other side.

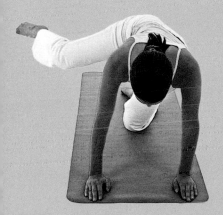

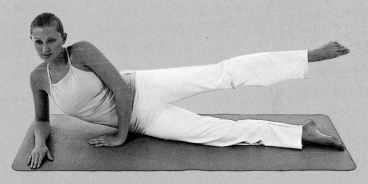

tabletop

Kneel on all fours, keeping your back straight and looking down. Raise one bent leg out to the side, keeping your weight evenly distributed among your hands and other knee. Holding the raised knee high, lift and lower in eight small pulsing movements, then swap to the other side.

Finish by bringing the raised foot slightly forward, so the leg is less bent, and make circles with the foot.

side lifts

Lie on your right side, propped up on one elbow. Make sure your hips are aligned one above the other. Slowly lift your left leg towards the ceiling and lower it, stopping just short of resting on the right leg.

After eight repetitions, change the movement. Bend the left leg when it's raised and bring the left knee forwards as if towards your face.

After eight repetitions of this, bend the left leg, bring the left knee down to the floor and keep it there. Raise the right (lower) leg, keeping it straight, and bring it down to just above the floor before raising it again.

help! I'm not losing weight

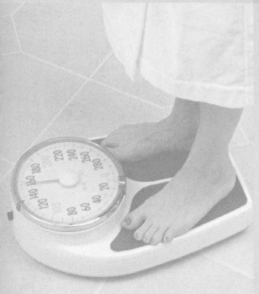

You're following the fat-loss plan faithfully and yet the weight is stubbornly clinging on. What's happening? Don't panic and launch into a crash diet – you'll ruin your skin and look dreadful on the day. You're almost certainly making one of the small mistakes that most people encounter. Do the Detox (see pages 114–115) or, if necessary, swap to the Superfast Diet on pages 118–121. You've left yourself time to get this right, so take a look at what you're doing and try keeping a food diary for a few days to see whether any patterns emerge. Start by asking yourself these questions.

dietary dilemmas

Have you hit a plateau? If you were losing weight steadily and then suddenly stuck, your body may have become accustomed to the smaller intake. Eat more non-starchy vegetables (anything other than roots such as potatoes), as research has found these fill you up better than fatty foods. Also try increasing your output through exercise. You burn food faster after aerobic exercise, and muscle building speeds up your metabolism. So add 15 or 30 minutes to your regular workout and watch the weight go.

Are you adding more extras than you think? You don't want to become obsessed with weight, and everyone needs an occasional indulgence. But if that's one or two every day, you're clocking up large amounts of extra, and probably empty, calories.

Do you skip breakfast? Scientists have found that people who eat breakfast are, on average, lighter than those who don't – possibly because they're not desperate for a doughnut at 11am.

Are you eating too much at a time? Look for a Diet Plate™, which is divided into sections showing how much to serve of different kinds of food. Or try weighing all your food for a week, to check. This could kick-start your weight loss, as you'll be tempted to put less food on the scales!

Do you eat out a lot? You probably know to look for low-fat options. But portion sizes have ballooned over the past few years. Research has

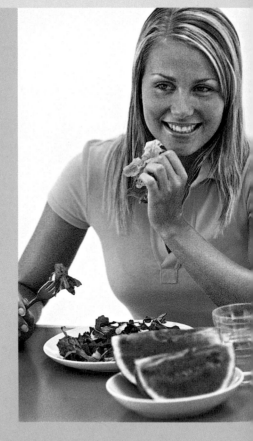

Above There's no need to go hungry. Choose from the huge variety of non-starchy vegetables to replace foods high in fat. Add some fresh fruit too, to keep your sweet tooth happy.

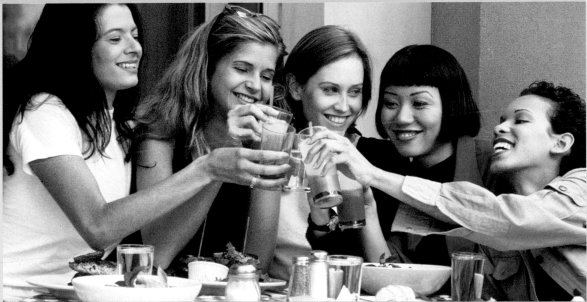

Above Time with your friends is precious – why waste it in an alcoholic haze? If you need a few glasses of wine before you relax with them, maybe you should find more enjoyable company!

found that people eat more from a large portion than from a smaller one, so ask for the smallest size.

Are you underweight already? If you're trying to make yourself unhealthily thin, your body will resist – it's fighting for your life.

Is it a hormonal problem? Hormones can play havoc with your weight, especially at eventful times like this. Your 'well-woman' clinic or gynaecologist should be able to find out and offer advice. Check also whether you have a condition such as an underactive thyroid or polycystic ovaries that could be making you gain weight.

Do you eat too fast? It takes a while for the brain to pick up the stomach's signals that it's full. When eating on the run, it's easy to take in more than you need before you realize.

Do you keep 'breaking the diet' and giving up? This isn't a diet, so don't feel you've broken it. It's just a way of eating healthily that happens to reduce your weight if you have any to lose. So instead of hating yourself and going on a guilt-driven binge, just accept that you wanted something else, and ate it. Then, if you choose, go back to eating the recommended way.

Are you sure you want to lose weight? Your fiancé loves you as you are, so why not do the same? If you can't resist your favourite treats, it's not worth making your life a misery. Relax and make the most of your curvy features, such as smooth shoulders and a beautiful bosom.

you are what you drink

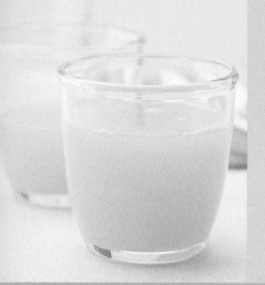

You've been eating healthily for three months. But are you counting what you drink? A common dietary mistake is to overlook the calories you're swallowing from a bottle, glass or cup. Most drinks contain little nutritional value. You may be unwittingly sabotaging each day's healthy eating efforts every time you quench your thirst. Alcohol is the biggest enemy, as it weakens your resolve not to overeat, as well as giving you a hefty slug of empty calories. But other drinks can also pack a calorific punch. So swap to healthier options till you raise your Champagne glass at your reception.

the demon drink

Alcohol is the big diet-killer. It is higher in calories than protein or carbohydrates, providing about 70–120 calories per unit depending on the drink. Your body also burns alcohol before other foods, meaning that those fatty snacks you nibble with a drink go straight on to your hips.

In the past a glass of wine or half a pint of beer equated to 1 unit of alcohol and about 85 calories, but measures and alcohol strength (ABV) have increased steeply since then. There are 150 calories in a medium (175 ml/6 fl oz) glass of ordinary red wine (12% ABV), along with 1.75 units of alcohol. So a large (250 ml/9 fl oz) glass of fairly strong wine costs you over 250 calories – and takes you over the recommended limit of 3 units a day. The stronger and sweeter a wine is, the more calories it contains. Luckily, a (100 ml/3$\frac{1}{2}$ fl oz) flute of 12% ABV Champagne is only 1.2 units and contains less than 100 calories.

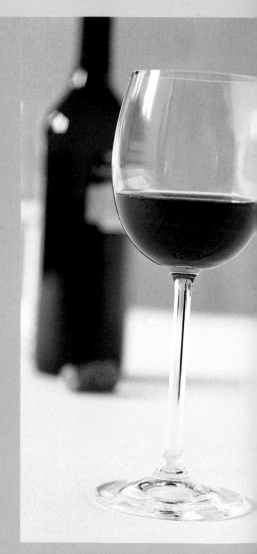

Strong beer and sweet cider top the weight-gain chart; mild beer and lager are better choices. Lowest-calorie spirits are gin, whisky, vodka and tequila at about 50 per unit, with creamy liqueurs around 80 per unit. Alcopops contain about 150 calories a bottle, on average. Syrupy mixers pile on calories, and in cocktails and punches you can't be sure what you're swallowing. Mulled wine is full of sugar: a medium (175 m/6 fl oz) glass of a standard recipe is nearly 350 calories.

Lightest options include mild beer (more drink per calorie), and spirits drunk with lots of low-calorie mixers such as mineral water, soda water, diet soft drinks, ginger ale or tomato juice. Wherever possible, look for low-alcohol or dry white wines, and drink spritzers made with wine and fizzy water.

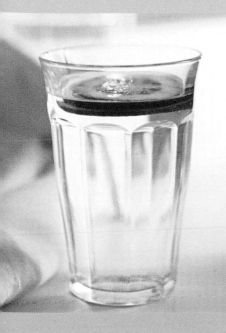

healthy drinks

Water (you knew it) is your best friend when you're trying to eat, or drink, light. It's a myth that you have to force 2 litres (3½ pints or 8 glasses) a day down your throat. But it's healthy, harmless, natural and unbeatably refreshing. And it's quite surprising what a lift water can give your skin when you start drinking more.

Herbal teas are another good option, offering various health benefits if wedding preparations start to take their toll, and something for every taste. Camomile promotes restful sleep, for example, and feverfew can ease headaches and migraines. Peppermint tea has been proved to calm indigestion, and ginger calms stomach-churning nausea.

Above Ice and lemon? Mineral or plain tap water with a slice of lemon makes a great thirst-quenching drink. At parties, avoid hangovers by drinking a glass of water for every one of alcohol.

Left A glass of wine no longer equals one unit of alcohol and 85 calories. Measures have increased so much over the past few years that it could be three times more.

naughty drinks

Soft drinks are a trap. Even those with artificial sweeteners often contain sugar, too. In the ingredients list, look for words ending in '-ose': sucrose, fructose and so on. They're all forms of sugar. Fructose is a naturally occurring ingredient in fruit, but when it's extracted and added to other products, it's just more sugar. Soft drinks also tend to contain a mass of chemicals you wouldn't really want to swallow if you thought about them, including artificial sweeteners.

Fruit juice is full of vitamins, but it's also high in natural sugars. Bought juices may contain added sugar, even if this isn't stated on the label. Try diluting fruit juice with water (fizzy water adds a sparkle) to subtract calories and be kinder to your teeth. Vegetable juices have a much lower sugar content. So-called 'fruit drinks' usually contain a tiny percentage of fruit juice along with water, sweeteners, chemicals – and, yes, plenty of sugar. Look on the label, where the ingredients should be listed in descending order of weight, largest first.

Tea and coffee are stimulants that don't do the condition of our skin any good. A few cups a day shouldn't do much harm, but skip the sugar and try to use skimmed or semi-skimmed milk – it's just as nutritious as full-fat. Aim to keep down to the two or three cups you'd miss most: for example, one when you wake up, a mid-morning pick-me-up and one when you come home. Replace the rest with water or herbal teas. When you're out and about, remember that a full-fat caffe latte packs a calorific punch, even without adding sugar. Choose the skinny option instead.

TURN TO DRINK
Sometimes when you think you're hungry, a drink fills the gap, so try a glass of water or some herbal tea first before raiding the fridge.

tummy-trimming food

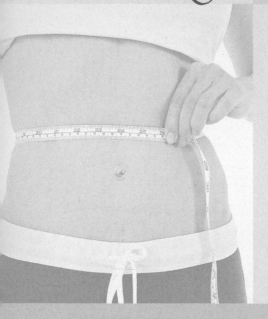

In despair because your tummy bulges despite 1,000 sit-ups? You may be suffering from fluid retention, constipation or wind (gas). A few dietary changes could see you looking sylph-like. For example, if you're drinking a lot more water than you want, in the belief that it's healthy, cut back to an amount that feels comfortable. Everyone's requirements differ, but most people need about 1–1½ litres (1¾–2½ pints) of liquid a day. But if you're not drinking too much, don't reduce your fluid intake. You may find that increasing it could even help your kidneys work better.

dietary changes

- Sodium grabs water and potassium lets it go. So cut down on salt (there's a lot of it in most processed foods) and eat more potassium-rich fruit and vegetables.
- Diuretics are meant to combat fluid retention by increasing urination, but they can make matters worse by reducing your potassium levels. Try the gentle alternatives opposite instead. If you do take any kind of diuretics, even herbal ones, check with your doctor first, and again if you notice any change in your health while taking them.
- Constipation is so common on a western diet, heavy in low-fibre convenience foods, that many people don't realize there's anything wrong. Changing to a healthier diet should help: less white flour, fat, sugar and salt; more fresh fruit, vegetables and whole grains. If your bowel still doesn't empty every day, try a different breakfast. A compote of dried fruit soaked in water overnight will gently stimulate your bowel, with some natural low-fat yogurt to encourage healthy bacteria.
- Sometimes your digestive system takes a little time to get used to a change in diet. Beans are high in fibre and potassium and low in fat, but they're notorious for producing wind. You can now buy harmless products that reduce this effect – ask in a pharmacy. Rinsing canned beans can also reduce their flatulent effects. A sudden increase in fruit and vegetable intake can also cause wind. This usually wears off as the fresh produce improves the health of your digestive system.
- If you eat too fast you're likely to be gulping in excess air, so slow down and take time to chew your food properly – both are easy ways to help prevent indigestion.

BEAT THE BULGE
Avoid:
- Salty foods
- High-fat products
- Highly processed foods
- White flour
- Artificial sweeteners

Have more:
- Potassium-rich foods, such as bananas, cantaloupe melons, oranges, avocados, spinach, cabbage and celery
- Live yogurt
- Hot water
- Charcoal biscuits or tablets

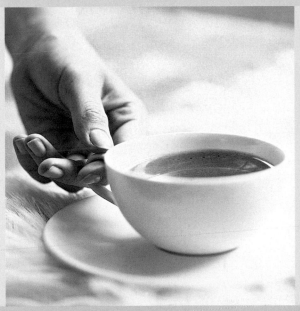
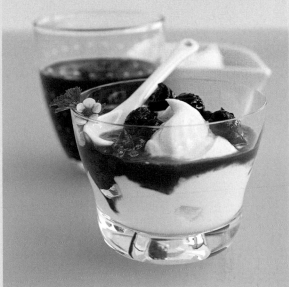

Above Slim down with simple, natural foods. A herbal infusion can gently reduce bloating, and a dried-fruit compote makes an effective and delicious remedy for swelling caused by a sluggish digestion or constipation.

combat bloating

Food intolerance may make your stomach swell, though it's not as common as you may think. If the suspected culprit is something you don't particularly need to eat, you could try giving it up for a few weeks and seeing whether you improve. Don't cut out whole food groups such as dairy produce or hard-to-avoid items such as wheat. See whether cutting down on them makes a difference. Keep notes of when the bloating occurs in relation to which foods, then see your doctor for referral to a dietician.

If your stomach is swollen with wind, drinking plain hot water can disperse wind amazingly fast. A simple tea made from aniseed, caraway, cinnamon or peppermint can often help, too. Alternatively, try massaging your abdomen with your fist with a firm clockwise movement, or try charcoal biscuits or tablets.

If you can't zip up your jeans till your period starts, your fluid retention is a form of premenstrual syndrome (PMS). Specialists such as the Women's Nutritional Advisory Service have devised entire eating programmes to combat this, including vitamin and mineral supplements (www.naturalhealthas.com).

liquid losses

If fluid retention makes your tummy bulge, try drinking tea, cranberry juice or a gently diuretic herbal infusion such as dandelion. Add some fresh dandelion leaves, celery and a few sprigs of parsley to your lunchtime salad, followed by a slice of watermelon.

FOOD COMBINING

Many people swear by the 'food-combining' diet, in which you eat high-protein and high-carbohydrate foods at separate meals. Most vegetables and oils are neutral foods that can be eaten at any time. For example, you could have a salad sandwich for lunch and a meat or tofu (bean curd) stir-fry with vegetables for dinner. It's a bit fiddly, but worth a try if you suffer from wind or indigestion.

a facial workout

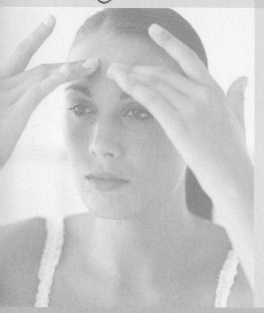

If months of poring over lists and sorting out problems are starting to leave their mark on your forehead, get in the habit of doing some brow-smoothing exercises. Evening is a good time, after you've cleansed and moisturized. Lubricate the skin with a little oil if you don't use moisturizer, and try to relax your face before you start. Look in a mirror to check you're working the right muscles. Don't drag the skin: it's the underlying muscle that should be moving. Press hard enough to move skin over bone, without hurting, instead of letting your fingers slide across your skin.

before and after

Start with some head and shoulder warming-up exercises (see page 10). Wake up your face by shutting your mouth and eyes tightly, then opening them wide. Purse your lips, then pull them back in a wide grin. Lean forwards and relax with head and arms hanging down. Do the head and shoulder exercises again at the end.

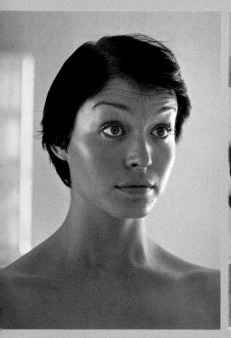
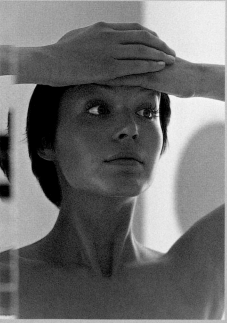

frown lines 1

Help reduce or prevent horizontal frown lines by working on the whole of the frontalis muscle, the muscle that runs across the forehead and raises the eyebrows.

Place your hands one on top of the other across your forehead and press inwards. Don't hesitate to press firmly, as the frontalis (unlike most other facial muscles) is attached to two bones. Raise your eyebrows as far as you can, resisting this pressure. Hold for 5 seconds, rest for a moment, then repeat four times. To relax the frontalis muscle, close your eyes and look cross-eyed for 5–10 seconds. Rest, and repeat three or four times.

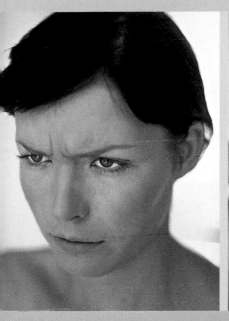
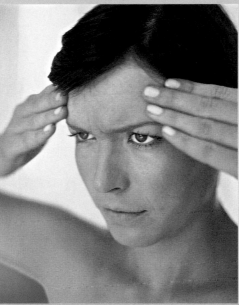
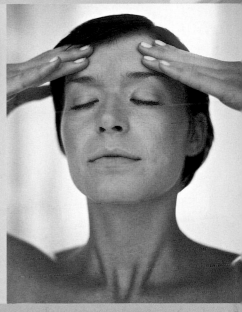

frown lines 2

This exercise works on the corrugator glabellae muscles, which create vertical lines between your eyebrows when you frown.

Frown tightly, then relax the muscles. Put the three middle fingers of each hand on the temporalis muscle (on the outer edge of each eyebrow) and frown again. Feel the pull on your fingers. Close your eyes and loosely shake out the muscles by vibrating your fingertips lightly over them.

> **TOP TIP**
> Put rosewater and sparkling mineral water in a spray bottle and spritz your face and neck when you're somewhere dry like an air-conditioned office.

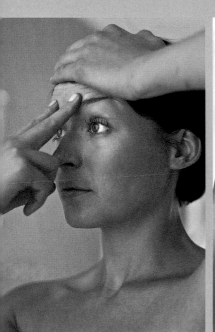
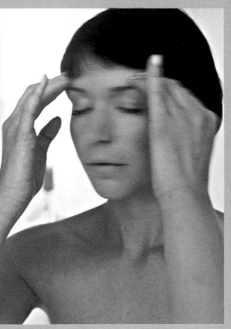

frown lines 3

This works on just the central part of the frontalis muscle, helping to reduce horizontal lines.

Raise your eyebrows, open your eyes wide and stare at a fixed point in front of you. Put the tips of your index and middle or ring fingers just above the eyebrows and raise the eyebrows against their resistance. Lightly press three fingers of each hand above the eyebrows and gently shake your head.

easy manicure

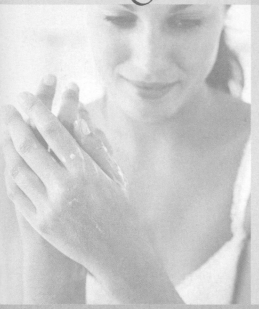

Don't forget that your hands will be the centre of attention when everyone crowds around to admire your wedding ring. As well as looking flawlessly manicured, they'll need to feel smooth when friends and relatives give them an affectionate squeeze. Classic photo close-ups include the bride and groom's hands, with wedding rings displayed, and of course cutting the cake. If, like most of us, you've neglected your hard-working hands, don't just buy rubber gloves for housework – make sure you use them! And start weekly manicures to ensure smooth and elegant hands on the day.

treat your hands

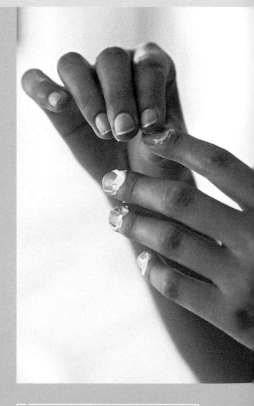

You'll need for the basic manicure:
- Nail brush
- Cotton wool and nail-polish remover (if you've coloured your nails)
- Nail clippers
- Emery board (wood file)
- Hand cream or almond oil
- Orange sticks (wooden cuticle sticks)

For a full-colour finish:
- Witch hazel or white vinegar
- Base coat, nail polish and top coat
- Cotton wool bud

1 **Wash and dry your hands,** cleaning your nails thoroughly using a nailbrush if necessary. Remove any sign of old varnish with cotton wool dipped in nail-polish remover, wiping from the base of each nail towards the tip.

2 **Clip your nails** so that you can just see the tops when you hold your palm in front of your face. Long talons are impractical and will give your guests an unwelcome jab. They may look spectacular on the day, but do you really want to have to avoid touching anyone? Nail clippers are the one sharp instrument you should allow near your nails, as your nails need to be cut cleanly.

3 **File towards the middle,** without whittling too much away at the sides. A wide oval is the classic shape, strong as well as elegant.

SCRUB YOUR HANDS
Every time you exfoliate your face, use some of the scrub on the backs of your hands, then hydrate them with hand cream.

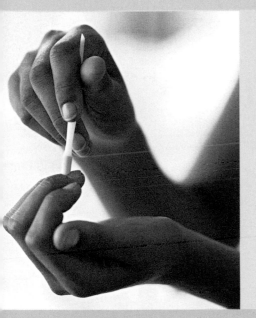

Above One layer of base coat is enough for a natural look, after nails have been prepared with oil and cuticles gently coaxed back into place. It also creates a smooth foundation for colour or nail art.

Left If overgrown cuticles are a constant problem, you can buy special cuticle cream to soften and tame them. Otherwise, use hand cream or almond oil.

TOP TIP
Even healthy nails can split and break if they're ill-treated, so shape them with an emery board rather than a harsh metal file, and stroke towards the centre.

---

4 **Soften up** if you're going to be putting on base coat or colour. Work some hand cream or almond oil into the nails, under their tips, into the sides and all over your hands. Leave it for a few minutes to take effect, then wipe off any excess cream or oil, wash your hands in warm water and dry them thoroughly.

5 **Push or lift overgrown cuticles back** gently using an orange stick, to reveal the half-moon at the base of your nails. Never cut your cuticles or use chemicals to remove them: you risk causing an infection and leaving the cuticles deformed.

6 **Massage with hand cream or almond oil** and finish here, if you're not going to paint your nails. Otherwise, wipe them with a little witch hazel or white vinegar if the earlier wash didn't banish all traces of cream or oil.

7 **Apply a fine layer of base coat to your nails**, your fingers spread out on the table. Work in one direction only, brushing from the base of the nail to the tip. For an elegant natural look, end here. Otherwise, let the base coat dry completely – this is vital at every stage for a smooth finish. Then apply polish with the same one-way movement and allow to dry. Apply a second coat of polish and allow to dry.

8 **Apply a top coat** and allow to dry, then wipe any stray polish off your fingers with a cotton wool bud dipped in polish remover. If you find this tricky, use varnish-remover pads or hold the cotton wool in tweezers.

dos and don'ts

Do...
● Use rubber gloves and barrier cream, and resolve to take at least as much care of your hands as you do of your hair.
● Buy the worst-tasting anti-nail biting preparation available, and paint it on your nails if the run-up to your wedding has you biting them.
● Stock the fridge with calcium-rich low-fat milk or yogurt to counteract weak nails that split easily.
● Adopt the habit of massaging hand cream or almond oil into your hands and nails every evening.
● Be patient enough to let each coat of nail polish dry completely before you start the next – the end result really is worth the wait.

Don't...
● Use a sharp metal nail file or cuticle stick on your nails, as sharp instruments can easily damage nails.
● Use a nail-strengthening base coat on weak nails for more than a few weeks at a time. Increase your calcium intake instead – see above.
● Leave nail polish on for weeks at a time because it can discolour your nails.

pampering pedicure

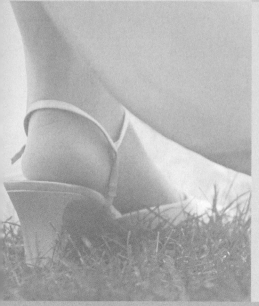

Like a facial or a manicure, this offers a chance of some relaxing downtime. Whether you're doing it at home or having a professional treatment, alone or catching up with your best friend, take the time to complete each step and enjoy the pampering experience. Ideally, you should get into the habit of soaking your feet in warm water and then exfoliating them, including the soles, at least once a week. Or add this to your beauty routine when you're giving yourself a body scrub. For a quick lift, dip tired feet alternately into bowls of warm water and cold water.

foot work

Assemble your manicure kit (see page 52), plus a nail buffer, a large bowl of hot water for your feet, a towel and a pumice stone. Sit in a comfortable chair within easy reach of a table: you're going to be there for a while. If you're alone, put on a favourite film or music or have a good book ready.

1 **Remove old nail polish** If your toenails are already painted, start by wetting a cotton wool ball with nail-polish remover and wiping off the polish, stroking from the nail base to the tip.

2 **Buff up** If your toenails are thick or ridged, gently smooth them with a nail buffer. Be careful not to rub too much away, as over-enthusiastic buffing can weaken nails.

3 **Enjoy a good soak** Wash your feet well, cleaning your nails with a nail brush. Then soak your feet for 5 minutes in warm, soapy water, and dry.

4 **Scrub up** Exfoliate gently using a pumice stone.

5 **Cut your nails** Cut or clip your nails straight across the top. You can round off the corners enough to stop them snagging, but leave them quite square so that the sides aren't at risk of ingrowing. Keep them fairly short, so that they can't be damaged by your shoes.

6 **Massage time** Massage your feet and nails using almond oil or foot cream. If you have any signs of fungal growths or infection, rub the area with tea tree oil instead. Buy an antifungal preparation from your local pharmacy if the problem continues.

7 **Banish cuticles** Push back cuticles with the orange stick if necessary. Wipe nails clean with witch hazel.

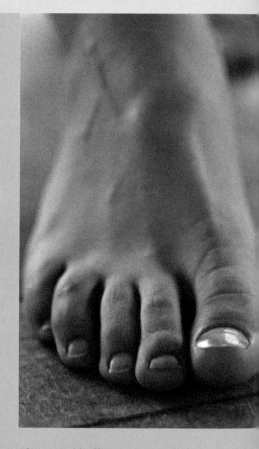

Above Nail buffers are too harsh for fingernails, as they can cause thinning, but they can give your toenails a natural healthy gleam without a hint of polish. Buff them gently to a light sheen.

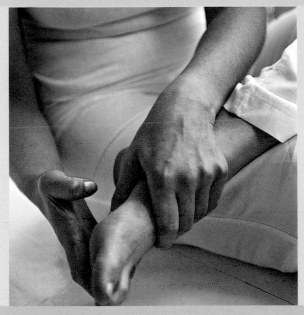 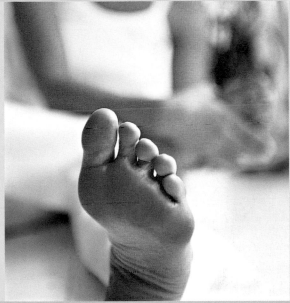

Above Our feet rarely get the kind of loving treatment that we lavish on other parts of our bodies. Take time during a pedicure to massage your feet, wriggle your toes, stretch them out, let them breathe.

8 **Spread 'em** Separate your toes with cotton wool balls, making sure no wisps of cotton wool stray on to the nails.

9 **Brush on the base** Paint on a base coat, brushing from base to tip. For a natural look, stop here. Otherwise, paint on a coat of polish and allow to dry completely. If it's even slightly tacky when you start the next coat, the finish will be messy and uneven.

10 **Top up the colour** Paint on a second coat and allow to dry, then paint on a top coat and leave to dry.

dos and don'ts

Do...
- Give your feet an intensive treatment every now and then. Wash and dry them thoroughly, then massage in plenty of foot cream or almond oil. Put on cotton socks and relax for the rest of the evening.
- Cut your toenails shorter if you go jogging, to prevent injury.
- Revitalize tired feet by soaking them for, alternately, two minutes in warm water with a drop of lavender oil, and one minute in cold.
- If your ankles ever look puffy, regularly massage feet and ankles with upward movements towards the heart.

Don't...
- Wear shoes that are tight or have excessively pointed toes. Apart from the long-term damage, feet that are regularly forced into an unnatural shape look ugly when they're revealed in sandals.
- Forget to dry thoroughly between your toes after a bath or shower, to prevent fungal infections.

TOP TIP
Match your toenail colour with your fingernails, buff your bare nails to a natural sheen or add a daring flash of scarlet for a tongue-in-cheek edge to all that virginal white.

perfect accessories

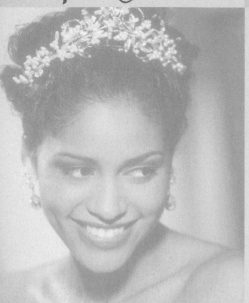

Your bridal outfit isn't complete without the right lingerie and accessories, so make enough time to find exactly what you want. Choosing a head-dress can be as enjoyable as choosing the dress, and can add a dazzling finishing touch.

Make sure you have at least one dress fitting wearing all your bridal lingerie. It makes such a difference that some dressmakers ask you to wear it at every fitting.

Check that everything goes together: head-dress with hairstyle with neckline with jewellery with dress. Although this sounds obvious, it's all too easily overlooked.

headwear

Like a hairstyle, the head-dress can complement your assets and disguise imperfections. A tall head-dress adds length to a round face; one with details beside your face adds width if your face is narrow. A simple head-dress won't distract attention from your perfectly honed waist, whereas a tiara will draw all eyes in that direction.

Remember the rule An elaborate dress calls for relatively plain accessories, whereas a classic sheath or empire-line will work equally well with either a simple or a dazzling head-dress. In general, an ornate head-dress is best complemented by a fairly simple hairstyle with few competing details. Fresh or silk flowers look perfect with most styles.

lingerie

Lingerie is the secret of a flawless bridal silhouette. It's worth going to a specialist supplier to find the perfect set: ask at your bridal shop if they can recommend anyone.

A better shape If you're wearing a strapless or off-the-shoulder style, try it on without a bra and see whether your silhouette is perfect or whether it would work better with some shaping. Full-busted brides should check how the dress looks, not only when they've just put it on, but after they've been wearing it and moving around for a while. Some styles lend themselves to sewn-in inserts, so ask the assistants whether that would be possible. Others look best with a strapless bra.

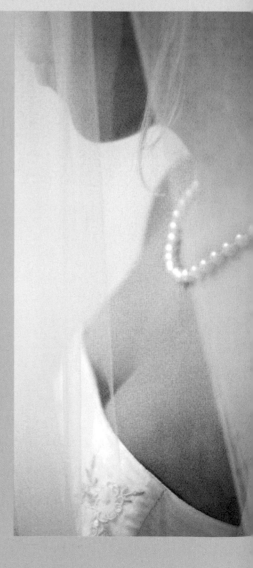

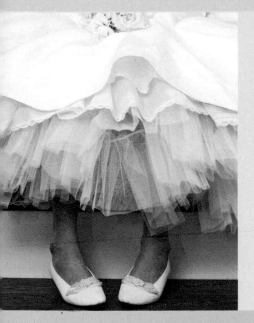

If your dress covers your shoulders, you have a much wider range of options. For the best fit and shape, have yourself measured by a specialist at a department store or bra shop. Take a few bras to try on during dress fittings, to get an idea what will work best. Take time to check that the shape of your underwear doesn't show through delicate fabric and straps don't creep into view as you move around. If you're wearing a fitted dress, get a friend to check from behind that there's no 'visible pantie line' even when you kneel or move.

Material girl The fabric of your lingerie makes a difference, too:
- Synthetic underwear can make your dress hang badly and cling in all the wrong places. It can even build up static electricity and shock anyone who touches you!
- Cotton lets your skin breathe, but may not provide a smooth enough surface for the dress to drape over.
- Silk is a classic choice, and lets your dress hang perfectly. A silk slip makes a smooth foundation for any dress and is indispensable if you're wearing something fitted.

Above Rings on your fingers, bows on your toes ... this is one day when you can indulge your footwear fantasies without any guilt. Wedding shoes don't even have to pretend to be practical.

Left The soft gleam of pearls against flawless skin is evidence that, when all the elements are perfect, nothing works better than classic simplicity.

jewellery

Wearing heirloom jewellery makes a beautiful link with family tradition, and you may need to organize some of your outfit around it. Long earrings or a necklace, for example, need space to hang without bumping into a collar. Conversely, small stud earrings look best with either a high neckline, a necklace or long hair. To show spectacular jewellery to its best advantage, any other accessories should be kept simple.

New pieces for the day give you more leeway with your head-dress and neckline, as you can choose the jewellery to match.

shoes

Your shoes may not be visible most of the time, but you'll want them to look as gorgeous as your dress. Practise wearing heels the same height as your wedding shoes till you move with a graceful sashay. Walk as slowly as you need to, and remember to keep your back straight and your head up.

You're buying these shoes for their looks, but remember that they have to be comfortable, too. Don't condemn yourself to a day of intense pain or you won't be able to dance at your own wedding. Oh, and check that you (and your fiancé) have taken the labels off your soles, or everyone will see them when you're kneeling at the altar!

TOP TIP
Put the balls of your feet down first for an elegant glide when you're walking in high heels.

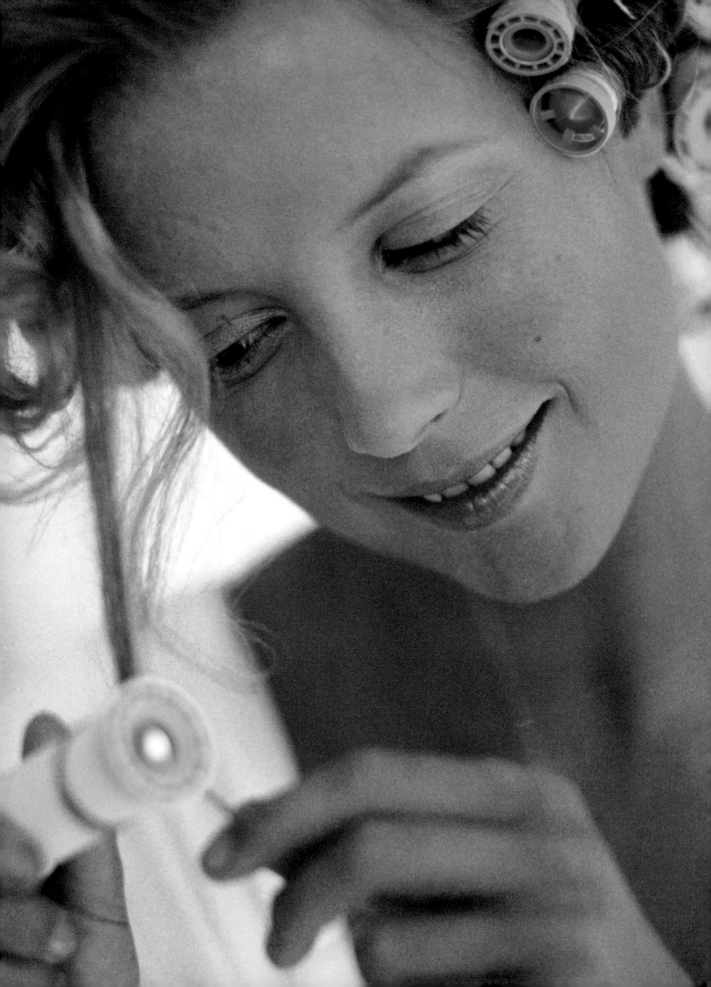

1 month and counting

*Following this month's plan should reduce tension and perfect your look. You'll be **eating to keep your energy levels high**, and following a gently detoxifying diet to deep cleanse your system, make your skin glow and reduce the appearance of cellulite. With your skin in beautiful condition, you'll be practising make-up that shows off your glow.*

*The exercises in this section will aid this process. Banish the lumpy effects of muscle tightness and fluid retention, and add height and lightness with **perfect posture**. In this final month, you can drop the muscle building and, if you wish, reduce your aerobic exercise, but still aim to work out three times a week. After warming up, do 30–60 minutes of aerobic exercise, then posture exercises from page 65, plus one or more of the body-sculpting routines from pages 36–43. Add The Cat stretch on page 61, and spend some extra time on your stretches to ensure a long, sleek outline.*

WEDDING PLANNING CHECKLIST: FINAL MONTH

- Chase any unanswered invitations, draw up the final guest list and make a seating plan.
- Finalize details and numbers with the caterers.
- Check that arrangements for your hen and stag parties are in place.
- Check that your wedding outfit will be ready, and have a final dress fitting with head-dress, shoes, jewellery and lingerie.
- Have a hair and make-up practice session, including your bridesmaids.
- Check that you've tried everything you're going to do in the final week to work out what to do and avoid risking an unexpected skin reaction.
- Be careful in the sun: don't risk sunburn or tan/strap marks that clash with your neckline.
- Check that your dressmaker, hair stylist, etc. will be available in case of last-minute needs.
- Confirm your final hair appointment(s).
- Buy single-use cameras. Delegate someone to hand them out, leave them on each table at the reception and collect them up afterwards.
- Organize wedding favours and decorations for the tables, if you're having them.

tension tamers

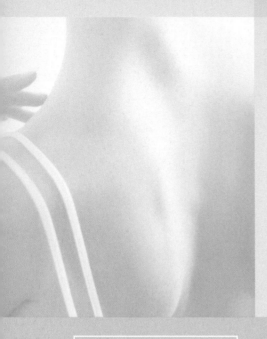

Even when you're coping admirably with wedding preparations, stress can make itself felt in your body. Your breath becomes shallow and your muscles tighten, inhibiting blood circulation. As well as causing headaches and increasing your risk of injury while you're exercising, tension makes you look hunched and bulky instead of tall and slim.

Take a five-minute break to do this breathing exercise and The Cat. If you can't use the floor, stand up to do the breathing exercise and the Flat-Back Lean. For tension in specific muscles, add the stretches on pages 11, 41 or 43.

BANISH TENSE MUSCLES
One of the best ways to unknot tense muscles is with a massage. Either book one with a trained massage therapist, or get one from your fiancé or best friend (see pages 92–101). Warmth helps, too, so try a sauna, steam room or warm bath.

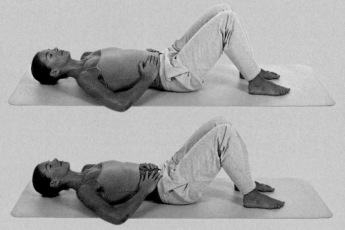

breathing from the abdomen

Lie on your back with knees bent and let your spine sink into the floor. Put your fingers on your navel and breathe in to the count of five. Aim to fill your lungs from the bottom so that your navel lifts, then fill the middle of the lungs and finally the chest. Breathe out to the count of ten, bringing your navel down to help expel air, first from the bottom of the lungs, then from the middle and finally from the chest. Repeat four times.

Variation: This can also be done standing, with shoulders relaxed and spine kept straight.
Note: If you start feeling light-headed, breathe in and out of a paper bag, or your cupped hands.

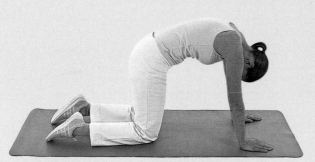

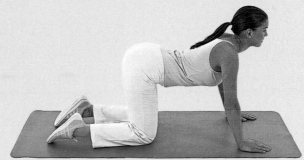

the cat

Kneel on all fours, with your fingers facing forwards and your neck and back straight. As you inhale, gently arch your back so that your navel dips towards the floor. Lift your head, leading with your chin as if trying to dip under a rope. Be careful to keep your neck long – don't let your head slump back and constrict the vertebrae.

As you exhale, round your back so that your head drops between your shoulders. Feel the stretch as you press gently upwards. Keep your abs and buttocks tight. Repeat the sequence four times.

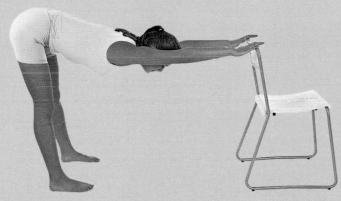

TOP TIP
Try yoga and Pilates, two exercise forms that create a long, lean physique by emphasizing stretching.

flat-back lean

The muscles around our spines store a lot of tension, especially when we're scribbling lists or thank-you notes with one eye on the time. This stretch will help ease them out.

Stand with your legs hip-width apart and lean down to hold the back of a table or sturdy chair, which your fingertips can just reach. Bend your knees slightly if you feel any strain in your lower back. Lengthen your spine as far as you can and let your head sink down to release any tension in the neck and shoulders. Hold the stretch for at least a minute, breathing steadily, and you should feel the spine extend further.

lymph boosters

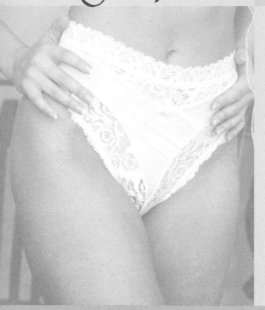

Fluid retention is the enemy of a smooth silhouette. Not only can it increase the size and lumpiness of the dimpled fat on women's hips and thighs, known as cellulite, it can also cause swollen ankles and a bulging stomach. On top of that, it can make your face look puffy and put bags under your eyes – not what you want to see on your wedding morning.

The exercises on these pages aim to stimulate the flow of lymph, which carries waste products from the body's cells. Do this brief routine three to seven times a week, first thing in the morning.

butterfly

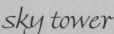

Sit on the floor with your back straight, your legs apart, knees bent and soles together. Rest your hands on your ankles with your arms by your sides. As you breathe out, bring your knees up to press against your arms. Press them back down as you inhale. Repeat ten times.

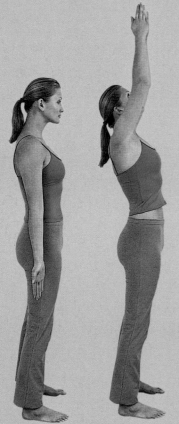

sky tower

Stand up straight with your feet slightly apart, your arms by your sides, stomach and buttocks tucked in and held firm. As you breathe in, turn your palms outwards, then raise your arms slowly out beside you and up above your head. Press your palms together, pointing your index fingers to the sky, and stretch upwards throughout your whole body. Hold for 5 seconds. Breathe out as you return to your starting position. Repeat five times.

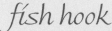

fish hook

Stand with your legs apart and feet pointing straight ahead. Breathe in, stretch out your arms beside you and raise them to shoulder-height. As you breathe out, drop your right arm to your side. As you breathe in, lift your left arm up beside your head, close to your ear, with your palm upwards. Keep your hips facing forwards and bend gently sideways. Don't tip forwards or backwards. Hold for 5–10 seconds, breathing naturally. Return to your start position as you breathe out. Repeat on the other side.

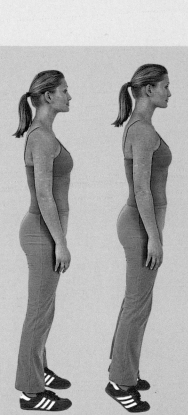

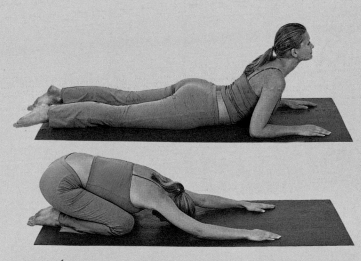

calf raises

Stand with your toes slightly turned in. Rise slowly on to your toes and return to your starting position in a smooth movement.

cobra

Lie on your stomach with your forehead on the floor and your hands under your shoulders. Keep your heels together and clench your buttocks. On an exhalation, roll your head gently up off the floor. On the next inhalation, lift your head, shoulders and chest off the floor as far as is comfortable. Keep your neck in line with your spine. On the next exhalation, lower your body and move your buttocks back, until you're sitting on your heels if possible. Relax in this position for a few seconds. Repeat the sequence three times.

On the last repetition, relax in the final position for several breaths and then slowly come up to standing. Your head should remain bowed as you do this and come up only when you are standing upright.

perfect poise

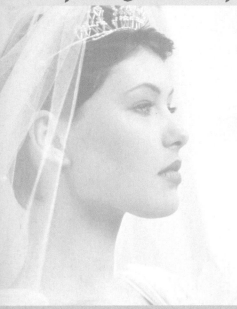

Good posture is probably the world's simplest beauty secret. It makes you instantly look taller and slimmer, with a lighter step, perkier breasts and longer limbs. Your movements become easier and more graceful; your clothes hang better. You take in more oxygen, improving your skin and creating a fund of new energy. You look and feel more alive, and you may even find that people react to you more positively as you radiate vitality.

All this just from standing up straight? That's the secret: most of us have the wrong idea about posture.

how not to stand

When we try to stand tall, we adopt a rigid military stance: chin up, chest out, shoulder blades colliding. We pull in our stomach muscles so tightly we can hardly breathe. Or else we copy models, thrusting the pelvis forwards to create a back-breaking arch in the spine.

Look in a full-length mirror, from the front and the sides – those found in changing rooms often give you a back view, too. Is your pelvis jutting nearly as far forwards as your toes? Is one hip higher than the other? Is one shoulder further forwards? Are you knock-kneed? Are your shoulders rounded, with your head either bowed or tipped back to compensate?

Most of us breathe too shallowly – yoga teachers often recommend drawing breath deeper down so it feels as if you're 'breathing into your stomach'. Don't worry that this will make your stomach stick out. When you stand tall, your lungs have more room to expand, so you can draw breath further down while still keeping the lower abdominal muscles strong and active.

Regular stretching (see pages 11 and 61) helps improve posture, as do exercises such as the Tension Hold (see page 40) and Back Curl (see page 16), which strengthen the core muscles.

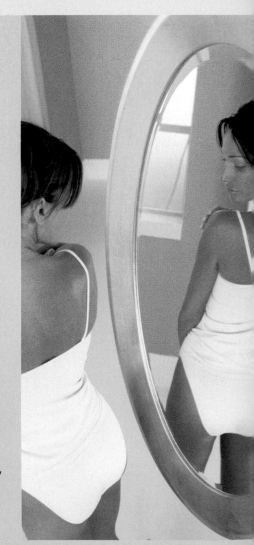

Right Take a critical look at yourself, not to denigrate your shape but to check if you've slipped into bad habits of standing or moving that don't do you any favours.

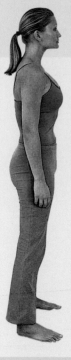

standing tall

Stand with your feet slightly apart, toes pointing forwards. If your toes turn out, your knees are likely to buckle inwards, destabilizing your whole body. Imagine you're suspended from a string at the crown of your head. Focus on pulling your body upwards, starting at your neck and pulling up through your chest to your waist and hips. Feel the gap between your shoulders and ears lengthening, and each vertebra spreading out from its neighbours.

Now focus on engaging your abs. Pull your navel back towards your spine without restricting the flow of breath into the area below your ribs. Imagine your pelvis is a bowl of water. If your back is arched, water will pour out at the front. If it's hunched up, water will spill from the back. Tuck your bottom in to keep the bowl flat.

Correct your posture every time you think of it. Put sticky red dots around your home or workplace and do it every time you see one.

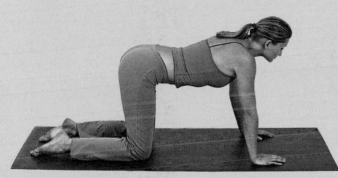

arm and leg raises

Kneel on all fours. Raise your right arm and left leg and stretch them out. Focus on using your core muscles to hold you stable. This is more important than your arm or leg movement.

Hold for 15 seconds and repeat on the other side. Repeat five times on each side.

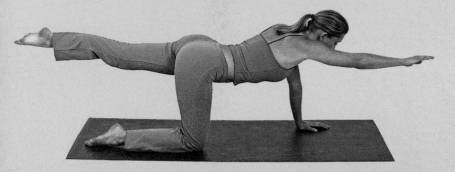

POSTURE-BASED THERAPIES
Any change in posture may feel strange at first. If it causes pain, you must be doing something wrong. An expert can solve problems quickly. Posture-based therapies such as the Alexander Technique and Feldenkrais can create graceful new habits in just a few sessions, so look for a practitioner in your area. Yoga and Pilates can help, too: ask the instructor to check on your posture.

juice cleansers

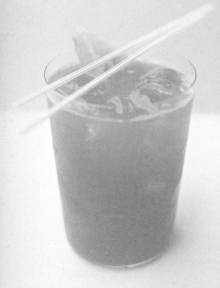

By now you should be around the weight you want to be, with clear skin and lustrous hair, and in this final month you'll be enhancing all your achievements. Even if preparations and celebrations have derailed your good intentions, there's still time. Start with the 1-Week Detox on page 115.

Either way, this month you'll be eating to deep cleanse your body, perfect your skin tone, smooth your silhouette and provide an extra boost of energy. Start with some delicious fresh juices – powerful sources of skin-saving vitamins, minerals and enzymes.

fresh fruit and vegetable juices

Juices can be bought, but are infinitely better made from fresh produce just before you drink them. You'll need a juicing machine – a blender or food processor mixes up the entire fruit rather than extracting juice, and anyway they aren't powerful enough to cope with raw vegetables.

Enjoy fresh juice as a snack, or as a meal replacement once a day. Try fruit juice for breakfast, or two glasses of vegetable juice for lunch. Apple and carrot are the classic mix, good when detoxing or any time, and an exception to the general rule that fruits and vegetables don't mix well.

Denser ingredients like avocado and banana turn a juice drink into a thick shake – higher in calories, but satisfying when you're hungry.

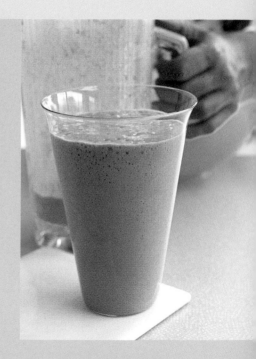

juice recipes

To aid detoxification Mix two parts of carrot with one each of celery, spinach and lettuce, and a little parsley.

To maintain energy levels Mix four parts of carrot with one each of fennel and celery, plus a little ginger.

To improve hair and nails Mix two parts each of parsnip, green pepper and cucumber with one part of watercress.

To improve skin One part each of potato, radish, carrot and cucumber.

For inner cleansing Mix equal parts of watermelon and strawberries.

To soothe skin inflammation Mix two parts each of red pepper and tomatoes with one of white cabbage and a little parsley.

After a workout Mix grapefruit, cucumber and a little lemon, and top up with sparkling mineral water.

MIXING YOUR DRINKS
Try each juice by itself before mixing, as ingredients such as watercress are surprisingly strong. Fruits generally mix best with fruits, and vegetables with vegetables – but experiment to find your own favourite blends.

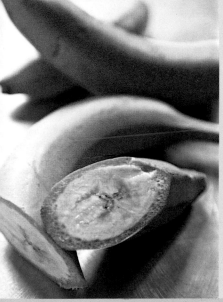

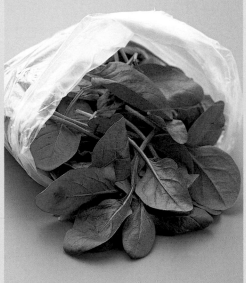

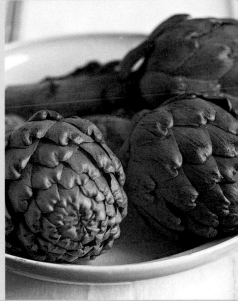

Above Bananas give a quick lift and make a drink more satisfying. The cleansing effects of spinach and globe artichokes could work wonders for your skin. Pick the freshest produce for the best taste and effect.

Left Many fruits can be put in a blender or food processor to make a thick, filling shake. Some, such as bananas and avocados, wouldn't work in a juicer and can only be blended.

WHAT TO JUICE

Apple Boosts the immune system and good for the digestive system.
Asparagus Strengthens skin and veins.
Avocado Good for the skin.
Banana Provides a quick energy boost.
Beetroot Cleansing and rich in soluble fibre.
Berries Contain powerful antioxidants that strengthen the skin.
Broccoli Packed with phytonutrients.
Carrot Good for the digestive system.
Cucumber A strong diuretic that also improves hair and skin.
Endive Counteracts stress and maintains a healthy colon.
Fennel Diuretic and detoxifying.
Ginger Rich in zinc and selenium, and adds a zing – use sparingly.
Globe artichoke Cleansing and diuretic.
Lettuce Rehydrating and protects the colon.
Melon (including watermelon) Cleanses and rehydrates.
Mint Freshens breath and rejuvenates.
Orange (and other citrus fruits) Good for skin, energy and circulation.
Papaya Aids digestion and is rich in vitamin C.
Parsley Freshens breath and maintains collagen.
Parsnip Diuretic and cleansing.
Pear Helps steady blood-sugar levels and prevent fluid retention.
Pineapple Aids digestion and may help heal collagen fibres.
Spinach Detoxifying.
Strawberry Energizing and rich in antioxidants.
Watercress High iron content helps prevent tiredness.

energy eating plan

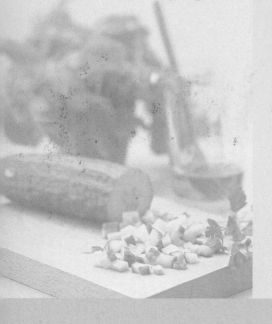

To support the work you're doing this month on increasing energy, try this 1-week vitality eating plan. Eating for energy involves always having a fruity or fibre-filled breakfast; eating protein at lunchtime because it creates longer-lasting energy, so is useful for counteracting the mid-afternoon energy dip; and eating more carbohydrates in the evening, to increase sleep-enhancing serotonin levels.

Like everything else in this book, these are meant as useful recommendations in an easy-to-follow form. Don't beat yourself up if you can't follow it in every detail!

	DAY 1	DAY 2	DAY 3	
BREAKFAST	Porridge with skimmed milk and a handful of berries. Glass of orange juice	Bowl of bran cereal with skimmed milk and a chopped banana. Glass of fruit juice	Fruit plate: an orange, a handful of berries, a slice of melon and a handful of grapes. Two oatcakes spread with a little ricotta or cream cheese	
LUNCH	Tuna or hummus sandwich on Granary bread. Salad of artichoke hearts, green beans, olives and tarragon on a bed of alfalfa sprouts	Chickpea Salad (see page 70), served with grilled king prawns, salmon or feta cheese	Salmon steak or omelette with tomato salsa, served with asparagus spears	
DINNER	Grilled portobello mushrooms sprinkled with Worcestershire sauce. Quick Lentil Salad (see page 70), served with spinach and broccoli	Spaghetti with pesto or Parmesan cheese, served with a large green salad, including watercress and baby spinach leaves	Bean or vegetable soup. Cheese on toast: two slices of Granary, soya or barley bread, topped with a little low-fat cheese and grilled	
SNACKS	A dozen almonds, peanuts or cashews. Two satsumas or a banana	Slice of toast with avocado and a dash of lemon juice. An apple or a kiwi fruit	An orange or a banana. A pot of low-fat yogurt with a little muesli	

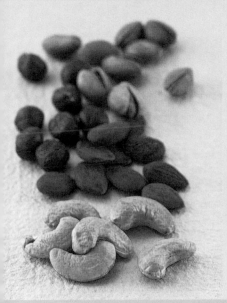
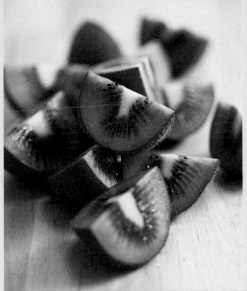
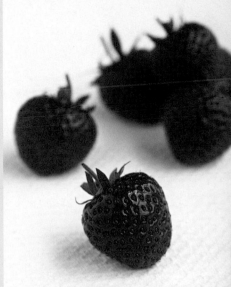

DAY 4	DAY 5	DAY 6	DAY 7
Pumpkin Seed and Apricot Muesli (see page 70), or a bowl of low-sugar muesli, with skimmed milk. Half a grapefruit	Low-fat natural yogurt with strawberries and apple chunks	Oatcakes topped with crème fraîche and blueberries	Poached egg with baked beans and grilled mushrooms. Half a grapefruit
Wholemeal tortilla stuffed with tuna or hard-boiled egg, plus bean sprouts, served with a salad of lettuce, cucumber, celery, chopped apple and walnuts	Mackerel or beans, served with a salad of beetroot, cooked leeks, chopped celeriac and grated carrot with a dash of horseradish sauce	Roast organic beef (fat removed) or Quorn™ or soya steak served with sweet potatoes, cabbage, carrots, peas and a little gravy	Stir-fried vegetables with tofu (bean curd). (Try bok choi, bamboo shoots, courgettes and mangetouts, with soy sauce, ginger and garlic)
Spaghetti bolognese made with 75 g (3 oz) organic or soya beef and a jar of ready-made pasta sauce with extra diced peppers and sundried tomatoes. Serve with dark-green cabbage or kale	Ready-made low-fat vegetable curry, served with basmati rice, lentils and spinach sprinkled with nutmeg	Cauliflower lightly steamed so that it's still crunchy, mixed with a small pot of cottage cheese, sprinkled with grated cheese and grilled. Serve with a green salad and couscous	Chicken or Bean Enchilada (see page 71), served with a large salad of red onion and red leaves such as chicory, lollo rosso and radicchio
A pear or a peach. A smoothie made from soya milk and yogurt blended with a handful of berries	A handful of pumpkin or sunflower seeds. Asparagus Guacamole (see page 71), served with two carrots sliced into sticks	A handful of nuts and raisins. An orange	Four celery sticks with peanut butter or cream cheese. A pot of low-fat natural yogurt with fruit. A pear or an apple

energy recipes

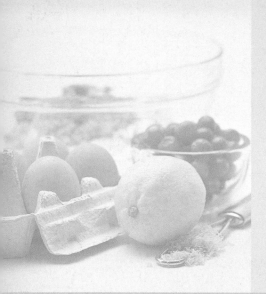

Use these well-balanced recipes as part of the eating plan detailed on the preceding pages. Or, since they're packed with ingredients that will increase your vitality and fill you up without weighing you down, why not try them out at any time during the period leading up to your wedding? Notice the quantities: most provide just one or two servings, for a quick meal at work or with your fiancé. The Chickpea Salad makes enough for two meals. But some things are too good to keep to yourselves – the enchiladas, for example, allow for a sociable evening with friends.

PUMPKIN SEED AND APRICOT MUESLI

SERVES 2

50 g (2 oz) rolled jumbo oats
1 tablespoon sultanas or raisins
1 tablespoon pumpkin or sunflower seeds
1 tablespoon chopped almonds
25 g (1 oz) ready-to-eat dried apricots, chopped
2 tablespoons orange or apple juice
2 small dessert apples, peeled and grated
3 tablespoons skimmed or soya milk

Put the oats, sultanas or raisins, seeds, almonds and apricots in a bowl with the fruit juice. This can be done the night before, if wished, and left in the fridge overnight. Add the grated apples, stir to mix and top with milk to serve.

QUICK LENTIL SALAD

SERVES 1

200 g (7 oz) canned lentils, rinsed and drained
3 spring onions, chopped
1 tablespoon chopped parsley
squeeze of lemon juice
75 g (3 oz) lean ham, chopped (optional)
salt and pepper, to taste

Mix all the ingredients together and serve.

CHICKPEA SALAD

SERVES 4

250 g (8 oz) dried chickpeas, soaked overnight
400 g (13 oz) cherry tomatoes, halved
4 celery sticks, sliced
50 g (2 oz) Kalamata olives, rinsed well and drained
4 spring onions, finely chopped
freshly ground black pepper
mint leaves, to garnish

Dressing
1 small bunch of mint, chopped
2 garlic cloves, crushed
200 g (7 oz) low-fat Greek yogurt
150 g (5 oz) reduced-fat hummus

Drain the chickpeas, rinse well and drain again. Put them into a large saucepan, cover with plenty of cold water and bring to the boil. Simmer for 1–1½ hours, or according to packet instructions, until cooked and soft. Add extra water if necessary. Drain well and allow to cool.

Meanwhile make the dressing. Mix together the mint, crushed garlic, yogurt and hummus.

Put the chickpeas, cherry tomatoes, celery, olives and spring onions in a serving bowl and mix well. Stir in the dressing, season with black pepper, garnish with mint leaves and serve.

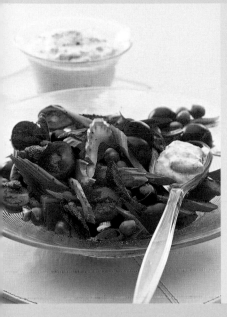
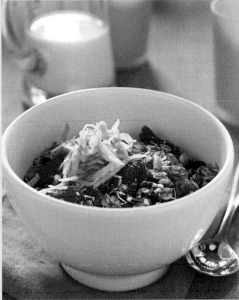
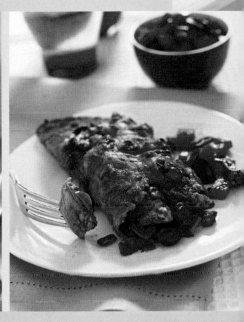

Above Left Chickpea Salad **Centre** Pumpkin Seed and Apricot Muesli **Right** Chicken Enchilada

CHICKEN OR BEAN ENCHILADA

For a healthy vegetarian alternative, try making bean enchiladas. Omit the chicken and double the quantity of beans.

SERVES 6

2 teaspoons olive oil
1 large onion, chopped
250 g (8 oz) canned pinto beans, rinsed and drained
300 g (10 oz) cooked organic chicken breast, skinned and cubed
4 green chillies, deseeded and chopped
1 teaspoon dried oregano
1 large tomato, chopped
1/2 teaspoon chilli powder
1/2 teaspoon ground cumin
400 g (13 oz) can tomatoes, blended
12 wholemeal tortillas
6 tablespoons tomato salsa
75 g (3 oz) low-fat mozzarella, grated

Heat the oil in a saucepan, add the onion and cook for about 5 minutes until soft. Stir in the beans, cooked chicken, chillies, oregano and fresh tomato. Warm through, then remove the pan from the heat.

Put the chilli powder, cumin and blended canned tomatoes in a saucepan and simmer for 2 minutes. Remove from the heat.

Dip each tortilla into the blended tomato mixture and set aside on a plate.

Fill each tortilla with 3 tablespoons of the chicken/bean mixture. Roll up and place, seam-side down, in an ovenproof dish. Spoon the salsa over the enchiladas, sprinkle with the cheese and bake in a preheated oven at 180°C (350°F), Gas Mark 4, for about 20 minutes.

ASPARAGUS GUACAMOLE

SERVES 1

75 g (3 oz) cooked asparagus spears
1 tablespoon low-fat crème fraîche
1/2 small red onion, chopped
a little tomato (optional)
squeeze of lemon juice
salt and pepper, to taste

Blend all the ingredients together in a blender or food processor and serve with vegetable sticks.

glowing skin

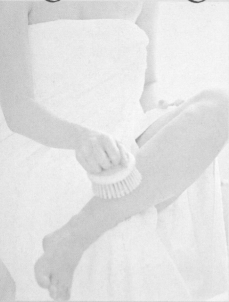

The most instantly satisfying element of a detox regime is the difference it makes to your skin. If you've given up a favourite stimulant such as caffeine, you may be feeling tired and headachy for a while – but your motivation gets a powerful boost when people start to notice the glow. It's not only a visible improvement: you soon start to feel your skin becoming silkier every day. Uneven texture starts smoothing out. If you're over 30, the benefits should be even more noticeable, as lifting and tightening effects reduce the appearance of any lines.

daily skin brushing

Speed the detox process by dry brushing your skin every morning. This does more than just improve skin condition. It's actually part of the cleansing process, which you're already carrying out on three fronts:

● Cutting down on junk food and stimulants
● Taking in healthier fruit and vegetables
● Improving your blood and lymph circulation with exercises

Brushing your skin continues the cleansing process by removing dead cells, while promoting the flow of lymph. It also stimulates the production of sebum, which makes your skin softer and smoother. The routine below takes a few minutes and can be done every day. For your body, use a firm brush made of natural bristles such as goat or boar hair, preferably with both a fabric strap and a long, detachable handle. For your face, use a very soft brush or a gently exfoliating cloth or pad.

If you've eaten or inhaled a lot of pollutants, your body has a heavy load to shake off, so you may briefly feel worse or notice a lot more blemishes on your skin while you're detoxing. If they persist, see your doctor and stop the detox.

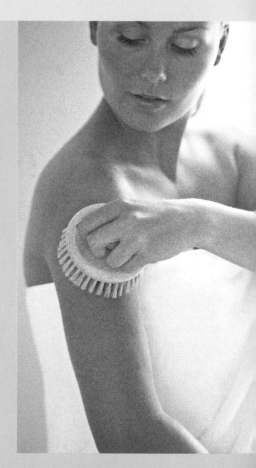

Above Brushing your skin feels strange when you first try it. But you'll soon come to love the exhilarating feel, not to mention the smoothness of your skin.

brush your skin

1 **Feet first** Rinse and dry your feet before you start. Brush the sole of one foot four to six times, firmly enough not to tickle, from the toes towards the ankles. Repeat on the sides and top of your foot, using long strokes that are firm but not hard enough to hurt. Work your way

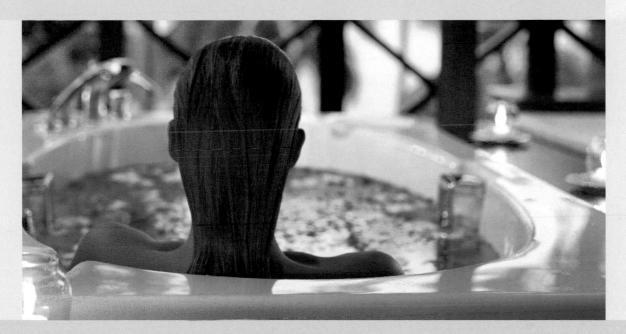

Above Not all detox ideas have an exotic heritage. Epsom salts are a traditional detoxifying agent that your grandmother may have used in her youth. Daydream your way back to a more leisurely era.

up the leg, finishing by brushing towards your groin. Repeat on the other foot and leg.

2 **Move on up** Continue with long, firm brush strokes up your buttocks and back. Brush in circles around your abdomen and then up your stomach and chest into your armpits. Work very gently on your breasts, with semi-circular movements from the nipples into the armpits.

3 **Handy work** Brush your hands and arms as you did your feet and legs.

4 **Face up** Swap to the soft brush to work very lightly on your face. Working from the centre of the face, brush outwards across your forehead towards the temples; down the nose; out across the cheeks towards the ears; and out along the jawbones.

5 **Wash it all away** Using the stiffer brush again, work down your neck, throat, upper back and upper chest towards your armpits. Finish by showering thoroughly to wash away any dead skin cells.

epsom salts

This is an evening detox technique, as it's likely to make you sleepy. Available from chemists and health-food shops, Epsom salts have a deeply relaxing as well as cleansing effect. Empty a packet into a warm bath (or use as directed on the packet) and stir until they're dissolved. Stay in the bath for 10–15 minutes, rubbing yourself briskly with a loofah or exfoliating sponge.

Have plenty of water to drink, and moisturize your skin before you go to bed.

You can do this once or twice a week, but not during or just before a period, as it can increase menstrual flow.

facial detox

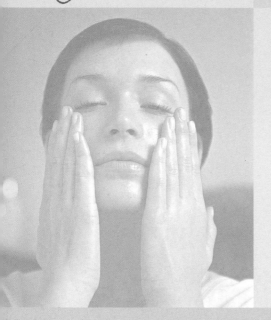

Manual lymphatic drainage (MLD) is a form of light massage that aims to stimulate lymph circulation. It is especially effective in reducing the puffiness caused by fluid retention. As a whole-body treatment, it is usually carried out by a specially trained massage therapist. But a simple facial version can work wonders in a short time. The following routine can be done every day while you're detoxing. Your throat may feel slightly swollen afterwards, which simply means that the lymph glands have been working harder. If the sore throat persists, see your doctor.

give your face a detox massage

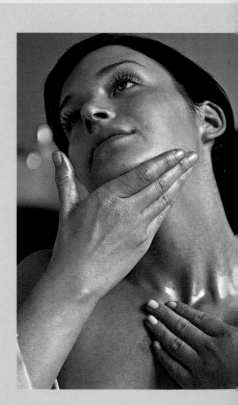

1 **Move on up** Rub a teaspoon of oil (see box) into your palms and apply to your neck and face in long, sweeping, upward movements. Then slide alternate hands up your neck to the jawbone, covering your entire neck from ear to ear and working lightly over your windpipe.

2 **Sideways moves** With your index fingers above your lips and middle fingers below, apply a light pressure before sliding your hands outwards to your ears.

3 **Firm pressure** With your fingers together and pointing up the face, apply firm pressure with your little fingers to the area beside your nose and mouth. Release the pressure slightly and, rolling your hands on to your cheeks, slide them outwards towards your ears, finishing with a firm pressure.

4 **The eye area** With the first two fingers of each hand, starting at the inner corners of your eyebrows, slide firmly out over the eyebrows. Following on from that movement, slide the first two fingers lightly inwards under the eyes.

5 **Cup your face** Close your eyes and, with your fingers together and using the whole of both hands, apply firm pressure to your face. Hold for a couple of seconds before releasing. Repeat to cover your whole face, from nose to ears and from chin to hairline.

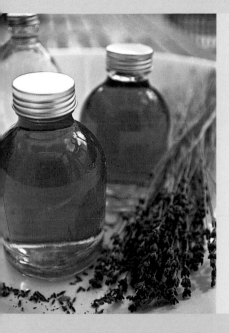

NATURAL HELPERS

Essential oils for massage that increase circulation and promote cleansing include cedarwood, cypress, black pepper, geranium, rosemary, orange and bergamot. Use one or two drops in a teaspoon of carrier oil, such as almond or grapeseed.

Herbal teas that help to improve circulation include any containing ginger, ginkgo biloba or rosemary. You can buy them ready-made in leaf or teabag form, or brew up your own by pouring hot water on a sprig of rosemary and a dash of grated fresh root ginger.

Facial massage will help to stimulate circulation at any time. Perform one quickly by gently slapping all over your face with the pads of your fingers and drum your scalp with your fingertips.

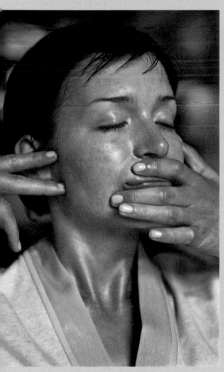

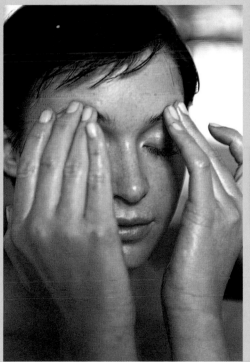

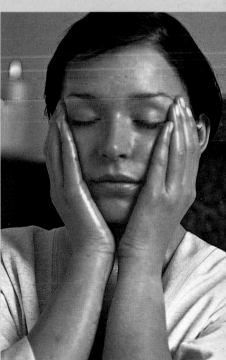

beauty masks

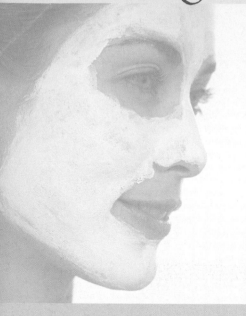

Planning a wedding involves seemingly endless journeys to caterers and suppliers. If traffic pollution and snatched meals have combined to leave your skin congested, deep cleanse with a mask made from ingredients you could find in your kitchen. A facepack – lighter and less penetrating – will revive tired skin quickly.

It is also possible to buy masks and facepacks ready made. Some moisturizing packs can be left on overnight, but don't do this unless the label clearly states that the pack is suitable to use in this way.

home spa treatments

Using any of the recipes below, mix the ingredients to a paste. Unlike factory-made products, these kitchen ingredients will vary slightly in texture and moisture content, so experiment to find a consistency that doesn't slip off your face or set too hard. They also contain no preservatives, so don't keep any leftovers. If you have enough of the mixture, cover your throat and upper chest, too.

Make sure your skin is cleansed before using a facepack or mask.

facepacks

Spread your chosen facepack mix on your face and neck, avoiding the eye area, and lie down for up to 20 minutes. Soften by dabbing with water, if you have oily skin, or milk; then gently massage off and rinse.

For blemishes Whisk an egg white until stiff, then mix in one teaspoon each of honey, fresh carrot juice and crushed garlic. Spread over spots and blemishes and leave for 20 minutes.

For dry or ageing skin Mash a quarter of a ripe avocado, then stir in a teaspoon of runny honey, two teaspoons of live natural yogurt and two drops of jasmine or rose otto oil.

For parched skin Mix pure aloe vera pulp or gel with a couple of drops of almond oil. When taking it off, wipe off any excess and then massage the rest into your skin.

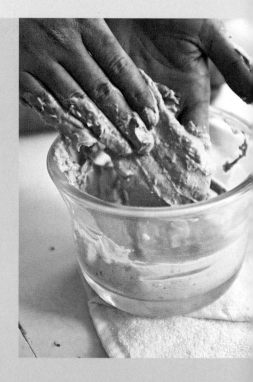

Above A nourishing avocado and honey facepack. The rich oils in avocado, the humectant qualities of honey and a dash of stimulating essential oil make this a rich treat for dry or ageing skin.

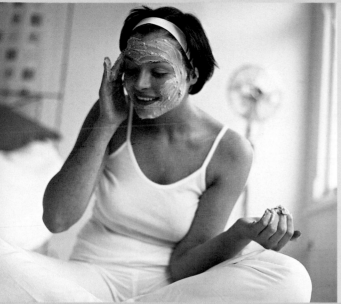 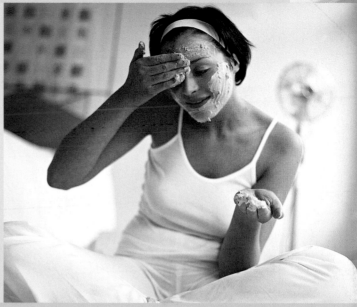

Above Be careful to avoid the eye area when putting on a facepack or mask. Not only is the skin delicate, but some eyes are sensitive to even the mildest products anywhere in their vicinity.

For oily skin Beat an egg white with the juice of half a lemon and an optional teaspoon of natural yogurt. If this is too drying the first time you use it, leave it on for just 10 minutes next time.

For flaky skin Mix a teaspoon of milk with two teaspoons of runny honey until well blended, and smooth gently on to skin.

deep-cleansing masks

A mask should be massaged well into the skin; its fibrous contents have a mildly exfoliating effect. Then lie down for up to 20 minutes. If a mask starts to feel too tight, take it off at once. Soften with milk or water, then rinse thoroughly without massaging again, as it will contain impurities.

Simple mask Mix two teaspoons of fine oatmeal with enough natural yogurt (for oily skin) or almond oil (for dry skin) to make a paste.

Revitalizing mask Mix a tablespoon of powdered brewer's yeast with a teaspoon each of natural yogurt, orange juice, carrot juice and almond oil. For oily skin, add a teaspoon of lemon juice, and for very dry skin, add another teaspoon of almond oil.

Clarifying mask Mix two teaspoons of ground almonds with a teaspoon of rosewater and half a teaspoon of runny honey.

Facelifting mask Mix a tablespoon of potato juice with the same amount of fuller's earth.

making up to the camera

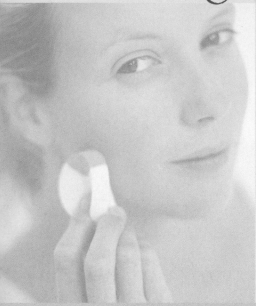

Bridal make-up is as much for the photo album as for the day itself. The classic look for a bride is light and fresh, with subtle use of colour: creams and pinks on fair skins, corals and peaches on dark complexions. This never goes out of style, and as it suits any kind of dress, it's the easiest to get right. But it's your wedding, and you may prefer something totally different – striking, glamorous or exotic.

Whether you're aiming for a traditional or an individual look, a few tips from make-up artists and photographers will help you shine in the best possible way.

suit your complexion

If you have oily skin, your natural dewiness may need extra control. Try oil-free foundation or oil-reducing gel to stop the camera turning your glow into a glaze. Finish with some matte powder even if you don't usually like it – it's invaluable for preventing the shine that cameras pick up so unkindly. Be careful not to create a heavy, unnatural look by overdoing the powder.

Dry skin needs the creamiest make-up at every stage: moisturizing foundation, cream eye shadow and swivel-up blusher sticks.

If you have dark brown skin, you'll need strong enough make-up to prevent your features vanishing as everyone's automatic cameras adjust for your white dress. Put on a little extra foundation, with concealer on any darker patches to even out skin tone. Use highlighter or cheek colour to emphasize your best features.

Any blemishes, including dark circles under your eyes, should be hidden with concealer. Use a shade lighter than your natural skin tone. To reduce high colour, try a green-tinted concealer. A yellow tint may be better at hiding brownish patches.

If you're pale and long for a golden glow, you may be considering fake tan. Try this out weeks in advance, and remember it will need to cover all your skin that shows. If you're unsure, just make the most of your porcelain complexion.

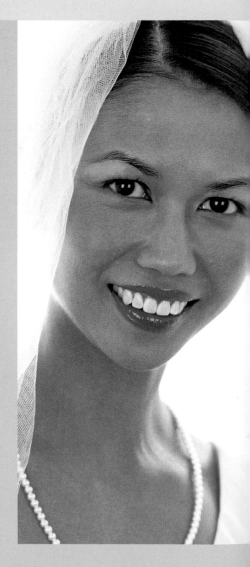

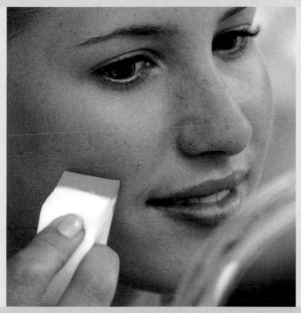

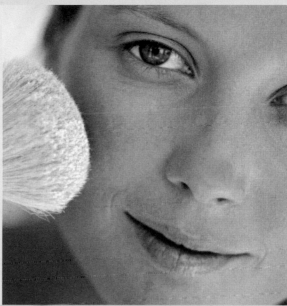

Above When you're buying a new foundation, try a little on your jaw line to check that the colour and texture match your skin tone.

Above right Invest in a large brush to apply face powder and a smaller one for blusher. If you have fair skin, soften the edges of blusher with a final sweep of face powder.

Left Whether your complexion is flawless or subtly enhanced with concealer and foundation, choose products that suit your skin tone for a fresh and natural look.

COVER UP

If you have a tattoo, scar or blemish that needs extra cover, look around for good camouflage make-up. Try as many as you need to find one that works for you and matches your skin tone. You may need several layers to cover a tattoo, but it can be done.

blusher

Softly sweep blusher over the apples of your cheeks. Use a light touch on pale skin. With a dark complexion, you can be bolder: try plum or rosy brown, or, on very dark skin, a rich bronze.

a lasting finish

One way of ensuring that your make-up lasts throughout a long day is to use both cream and powder versions. Start with foundation and concealer, cream blusher and eye shadow. Then put on face powder, powder blusher and powder eye shadow. Try this in advance to see whether it works for you. Otherwise, take 20 minutes out to redo your make-up for the evening.

face the camera

Whatever make-up you're planning, work on it as part of the whole look. At your make-up practice sessions, style your hair the way it's going to be on the day, and wear a top that's a similar colour to your dress. Make a simple version of your head-dress and have your jewellery at hand to try on.

Take some photos at your practice sessions, and use a make-up technique only when you're sure you've got it right. Don't be tempted by shimmery products and frosted finishes, for example, as they'll reflect the flash of every camera in the room. Light-reflective make-up and concealer, on the other hand, will help create a flawless finish.

photo-perfect features

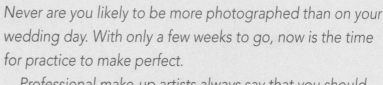

Never are you likely to be more photographed than on your wedding day. With only a few weeks to go, now is the time for practice to make perfect.

Professional make-up artists always say that you should emphasize either the lips or the eyes, but not both. Given that you may be wearing an elaborate neckline, head-dress, earrings and necklace, your make-up needs to complement your outfit rather than compete with it. At the same time, you don't want your face to vanish behind your veil. Follow the tips below for perfect photos.

luscious lips

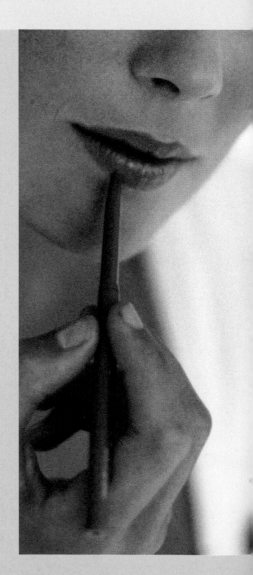

1 **Start with the perfect base** Before you even think about lipstick, exfoliate your lips with oat bran and honey. Gently brush off any flakes with a soft toothbrush dipped in water. Follow with lip moisturizer.

2 **Plump up those lips!** A dab of lemon juice may help your lips look fuller. A make-up artist can create a pout by taking lip liner and colour beyond the natural edge of a thin mouth, but unless you're very expert at this, be wary of trying it at home. Little slips that your guests will happily overlook will blaze out from your wedding album.

3 **Define your lip line** If you're using lip liner, match it closely to your lipstick. A dark line around the mouth shows up very harshly in photos. Apply your lipstick with a lip brush: this makes it much easier to follow the natural lip line, and creates a softer look.

4 **Use colour for warmth** A traditional warm pink or soft red lip colour will accentuate the freshness of a white or ivory dress. Bear in mind that neutral shades that look fine in the mirror may look too pallid in photographs. If you have dark brown skin, enhance it by choosing a lip colour similar to that inside your lower lip.

5 **Give lips staying power** Build up colour in layers for fuller-looking lips that will also hold their colour throughout the day. First apply lip balm, then liner, followed by a rich, creamy lipstick, which you'll need to blot and reapply a couple of times. Add a light coating of translucent powder if you wish, then complete with lip gloss or sealant.

6 **Kiss-proof lips** If you're not using sealant, finish by putting your index finger in your mouth and slowly pulling it out. Any loose lipstick will go with it, instead of on to the next person you kiss.

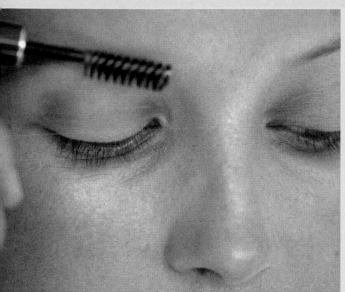

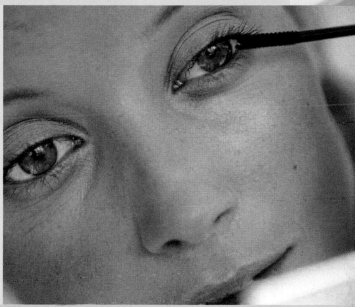

Above Brushing mascara down first, on the upper eyelashes, then upwards gives lashes a lift and makes your eyes look wide and sparkling. Just brush downwards on the lower lashes.

Left Liner can give lips a more clearly defined shape. Choose one that's as near as possible to the colour of your lipstick, and keep it sharpened for a flawless edge.

lustrous eyes

1 **Look natural** This is your day, so don't feel constrained to follow advice that conflicts with what you really want. But if you're aiming for that classic look, go for light (not white) eye shadow on fair skin, or a shade close to your natural colour if you're darker.

2 **Wide-eyed and gorgeous** Eyelash curlers magically widen your eyes. Complete the effect with a couple of layers of mascara – first downwards, then upwards on the upper lashes, and side to side on the lower ones. Comb the lashes if necessary to prevent clumping.

3 **Put a sparkle in your eyes** Black eyeliner is out, except on dark skin, as it creates a harsh effect against fair skin in photos. But a touch of white eyeliner on the lower lid will make your eyes sparkle.

4 **Staying power** Make sure everything's waterproof! The music or the sight of your grandparents holding hands may bring tears to your eyes.

VISUAL AIDS

● Looking great in glasses calls for meticulous attention to detail. The lenses make your eyes look bigger, but any make-up mistakes will be equally magnified. Flawless eyeliner and neatly combed lashes will give the look you want.

● If you're going without your glasses, you'll need to adjust your make-up. The strong colours that show off your eyes may look overpowering. If you're using contact lenses, they may make your eyes more sensitive. Avoid lash-lengthening mascara and any other cosmetic that could deposit a speck behind the lens.

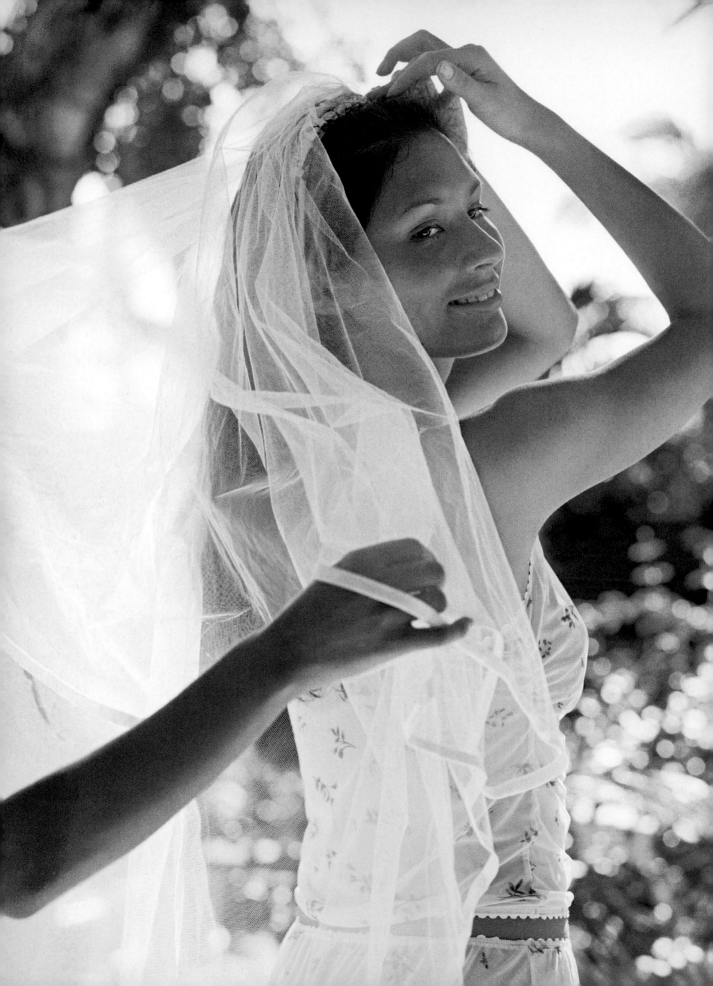

1 week to go

With a week to go before the wedding, schedule in some time to **relax and complete your beauty preparations**. Whatever you're doing, try to get out at least once a day for some fresh air. And factor in some fun with your fiancé and with friends, whether dancing, watching an escapist film or spending the afternoon at a beauty salon.

Drink plenty of water during this week, and don't use any product that you haven't already tested – the last thing you want is a skin rash. The only new 'treatments' in this week's plan are **massages** to soothe away any tension (see pages 92–101). For convenience, most of these massages can be done without oil (see page 92). You do need oil if your hand is going to move over the skin while applying pressure, as oil protects the skin and facilitates long, deep strokes. And a foot massage feels best with oil, which is why it's convenient to include it during the pedicure.

WEDDING PLANNING CHECKLIST: 1 WEEK

- Reconfirm photographer, flowers, cars, band and DJ.
- Reconfirm numbers with your caterer.
- Make final checks on your honeymoon booking.
- Pack for the honeymoon – and check that your fiancé has, too.
- Arrange for the cake to be delivered to the reception venue.
- Make sure that the best man has arranged for the hired outfits to be returned on time.
- Ensure that your outfit and everything else is complete and ready.
- Practise walking in your dress, and make sure your helpers know how to arrange the train.
- Wear in your wedding shoes around the house.
- Have a final hair and make-up practice, with your bridesmaids.
- Remind your groom to have a final trim at the hairdressers.
- Hold a dress rehearsal with the wedding party.
- If you're going to the wedding in a friend's car, get the driver to ensure that there's nothing that could catch the dress or leave a mark on it as you step in or out.

every morning

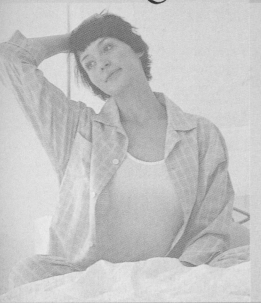

If everything has gone according to plan, this will be a peaceful week of relaxing massages and final beauty treatments. But when did any wedding go like clockwork? You've probably had to make some changes along the way, and still have some bits and pieces to sort out. Whether or not you're still busy, it's important to give yourself some time for relaxation during these final few days.

If everything's well in hand and you don't have to get up early for work, switch the alarm clock off one morning, catch up on sleep and give yourself a lazy start.

positive awakening

If there's anything other than relaxing music on the radio when you wake up, turn it off. Spend a few minutes with your eyes shut, enjoying the comfort of your bed and visualizing the day ahead with a sense of pleasant anticipation. If you have anything challenging to do, see yourself going through it in detail, step by step, and completing it successfully. Savour the feeling of satisfaction.

Have a long, comfortable stretch before you sit up. Then drink some water or herbal tea.

gathering energy

● **On Monday, Wednesday and Friday** (for a Saturday wedding), start with some stretches (see page 11), focusing on any part of your body that feels tired or tight, then do the Yoga Balance (see opposite).
● **On Sunday, Tuesday and Thursday**, do a 40-minute workout: a warm-up (see page 10), 20 minutes of aerobics (see pages 12–15), 10 minutes body sculpting (see pages 36–43) and some long stretches (see page 11). Finish with the Revitalizing Stretch opposite.

Whichever routine you followed, move on to do a few minutes skin-brushing (see page 72). Then take a shower and try to finish with a blast of cold water. You should now be feeling wide awake, relaxed and alert – ready for anything.

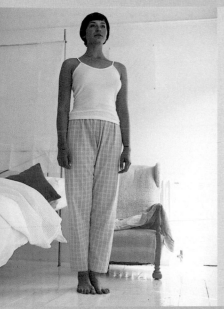
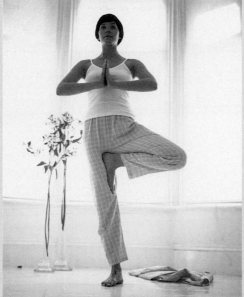
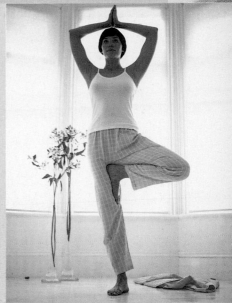

yoga balance

Stand straight with your shoulders relaxed. With your right foot flat on the floor, rise onto the toes of your left foot. If you feel steady enough, bring your left foot up to rest on your right calf or thigh, without pressing on the right knee. If you're feeling wobbly, put your toes back on the ground.

Raise your hands into the prayer position in front of your chest. If you wish, raise them above your head. Find a position you can hold for several breaths. Then repeat on the other leg.

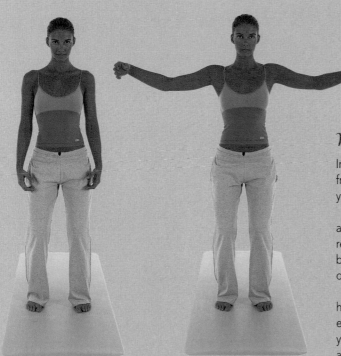

revitalizing stretch

Imagine yourself at the beach taking a break from your daily routine. Feel the fresh air that you're breathing.

Stand straight with your feet hip-width apart, abdominal muscles engaged and shoulders relaxed. Lift your arms to the sides as you breathe in; let them float down as you breathe out. Keep your shoulders down.

With each in-breath, lift your arms a little higher, feeling their strength and energy. On the eighth breath they should be stretched above your head, palms facing in. Turn your palms out as you lower your arms.

every evening

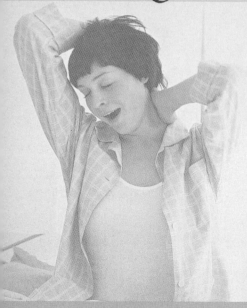

Whatever you have or haven't got done today, empty your mind. Let go of it. At this stage every bride could find something to worry about, from the seating plan to whether she really wants to be married! Don't let these natural last-minute nerves take their toll on your happiness and wellbeing. The thoughts you have when you're lying awake are unproductive. Create a relaxing routine to soothe away the day's concerns and ensure a peaceful night of refreshing slumber. This is a good time to share soothing massages with your fiancé: a tranquil way to help you sleep.

meditation

When you finish the day's work, sit in a quiet place and spend 10–20 minutes in meditation – a proven form of stress relief that also helps you organize yourself more effectively.

Sit either on the floor with your legs crossed or in a straight-backed chair with your feet flat on the ground or on a footstool. Fold your hands in your lap and shut your eyes. Feel your breath settling into its natural rhythm. Your mind will keep trying to distract you with thoughts and ideas; don't worry about this – just don't pay any attention to them and they'll eventually drift away. You may wish to set a timer before you start. Switch your phone over to the answering machine, too.

Start silently counting breaths: 'one' at the end of the first out-breath, 'two' at the end of the second and so on up to ten. Then start again from one.

Don't get stressed about trying to do this perfectly. When you lose concentration – as everyone does – simply bring your attention back to your breath and start counting again from one.

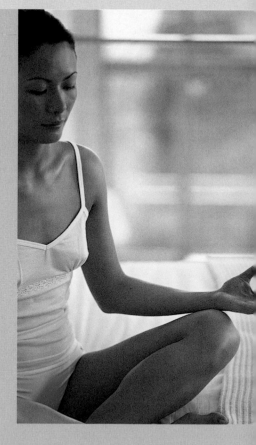

Above Meditation was traditionally done sitting on the floor. If you do this, find a comfortable position in which you can sit for 10 or 20 minutes with your back straight, giving your lungs room to expand.

mindful walking

After dinner, take a walk in the park or around your neighbourhood. Don't hurry, and try not to think about anything except what you observe as you go along. Make a point of noticing one new thing that you like each day: the texture of bark on a tree, the smell of wild buddleia, the sound of people sharing a joke. Try to keep this feeling of relaxed appreciation.

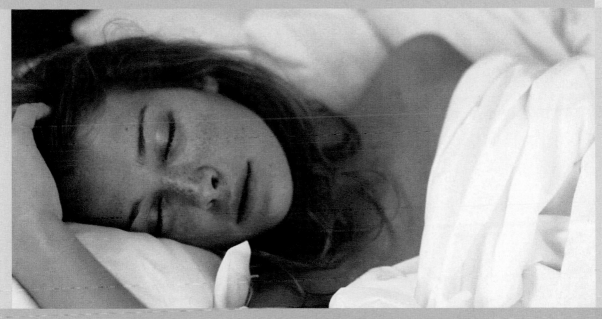

Above We really do need eight hours sleep a night to be in full health, though our busy lives mean few of us manage it. Recent evidence shows that a lack of sleep can cause weight gain by affecting hormones.

beauty sleep

The week before your wedding is the time you're most likely to be losing sleep – and the time you most need it! If you're not sleeping for seven to eight hours most nights, your skin tone and energy levels may pay the price.

No matter how busy you are with last-minute preparations, give yourself at least an hour to wind down in the evening. Listen to gentle music, relax with your fiancé, prepare the things you need for the next day – whatever puts you in the mood for sleep. Being too hot can stop you sleeping, so make sure your evening bath is no more than warm. If you're having trouble sleeping, a few simple changes should help:

● Don't use any kind of stimulant after 6pm. Caffeine, alcohol and nicotine will all keep you awake.
● Avoid anything that winds you up in the evening, whether it's a horror film, arguments or late-night news.
● Eat your last meal at least 4 hours before you go to bed.
● Just before you go to bed, have something that encourages your body to produce sleep hormones, such as a banana or a milky drink.
● Exercise in the morning or at lunchtime, not in the evening.
● It's hard to sleep when your brain's still active. Clear your mind by doing the breath-counting meditation (see opposite).
● If you wake in the night, don't lie in bed for more than 10 minutes. Get up and do something simple like cleaning shoes or laying the table for breakfast, then go back to bed.
● Try a herbal tea such as camomile or one of the commercial brands containing a blend of mildly sleep-inducing herbs.

7 days to go

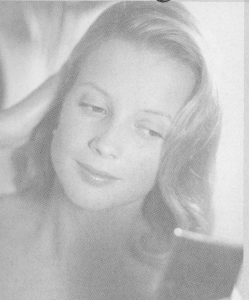

Today is the day for a hair and make-up dress rehearsal for you and your bridesmaids. Have your last pre-wedding appointment with the hairdresser by today at the latest, if you're having a cut, highlights or colour. From here on, just wash and condition your hair normally. Don't be tempted to do deep conditioning or any chemical treatments this close to the wedding. You can over-treat your hair, causing a lank or lifeless appearance. If you've been growing your hair, check that it's long enough for your intended style; if not, choose another style that works with your head-dress.

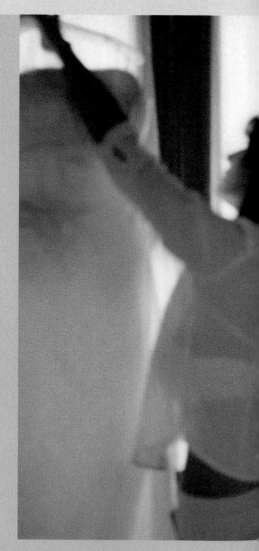

PLAN OF ACTION: 7 DAYS TO GO
- Every Morning routine (see page 84).
- Have your last pre-wedding hair appointment.
- Have a full hair, make-up and dress rehearsal for you and your bridesmaids.
- Rehearse the ceremony with all the main participants present.
- Every Evening wind-down (see page 86).

hair and make-up rehearsal

Position mirrors for an all-round view, and have someone taking photos or a video – something played back on screen at once would be ideal.

Wear a top of an appropriate colour and with a similar neckline to your dress. First do your hair, aided by your bridesmaid or designated helper. Put on the head-dress, and adjust your hair as necessary. Look at yourself from all directions, including a back view.

Then do your full make-up, preferably in the same kind of light you'll be in on the day. This is where you need friends or relatives who love you enough to tell you the painful truth. You don't want your look spoiled by a technique or colour that you've clung to long after it stopped suiting you, so ask them to be perfectly honest. 'Something old' should be a keepsake, not your eye shadow colour.

The bridesmaids' make-up should be unobtrusive and, without trying to look like clones, they should fit in with each other and with you. You don't want to be followed by a goth or a disco queen – unless that's the wedding theme you've chosen.

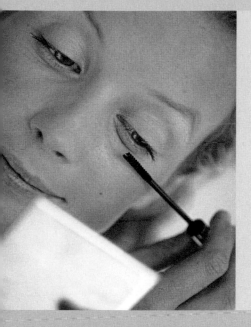

MENU: 7 DAYS TO GO

Breakfast Wholegrain cereal with skimmed milk and dried fruit, Granary toast with yeast extract, a glass of apple juice.
Lunch Grilled chicken breast, Quorn™ or soya steak, served with a mixed green salad.
Dinner Lasagne made with lean or vegetarian mince, served with courgettes, green and red peppers.
Snacks A fruit smoothie made with yogurt, kiwi fruit, oranges and berries.
Before bed Eat some fruit or drink a glass of orange juice and yet more water – to clear your skin.
Drinks Drink as much sparkling or still water as you can throughout the day.

Above Put on your full make-up and show it to close friends, in the same kind of light you'll be in on the day. This is your chance to do any necessary fine-tuning, so you can breeze through it next week.

Left An exciting moment: for the first time, you'll be wearing your wedding outfit and moving through the ceremony with the other participants around you.

dress rehearsal

If you're not wearing your wedding dress at the ceremony rehearsal, this would be a good time to practise with the bridesmaids, before you start putting on make-up. They need to know when and whether to hold the train, and practise walking in step with you. Ideally, play the music you've chosen for your entrance and exit so you can all learn to walk in time to it without looking unnatural.

You should also make sure you've practised walking, sitting and going up or down stairs in your dress, as well as standing. Stairs especially need a graceful technique for holding the skirt clear of your feet. Use the handrail: you'll be wearing an encumbering dress and unfamiliar shoes, so don't risk landing in a heap at the foot of the stairs.

If you'll be carrying anything other than your bouquet, make sure you can cope with them gracefully and practise handing them over to your chief bridesmaid when it's time to exchange rings. Is your dress a perfect fit now? If you've lost a lot of weight, it may turn out to be slightly longer as well as looser.

ceremony rehearsal

When you have the ceremony rehearsal, make sure the entire wedding party and everyone involved is there. Go through all the moves you will make, so no one is caught out on the day. Check that nothing has been misunderstood: one bride asked her church organist for the theme from *Robin Hood*, then had to stumble down the aisle, not to the romantic strains of 'I do it for you', but to the bouncy but rather inappropriate tune of a long-ago children's TV series!

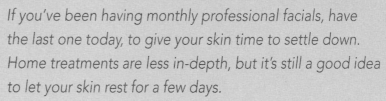

6 days to go

If you've been having monthly professional facials, have the last one today, to give your skin time to settle down. Home treatments are less in-depth, but it's still a good idea to let your skin rest for a few days.

Yesterday's rehearsals should have revealed whether you need to make any changes. Make a few notes of anything you noticed yesterday that you still need to perfect, and try to get it done today. This is the moment to do final beauty checks, leaving yourself time to make corrections and adjustments with professional help lined up if necessary.

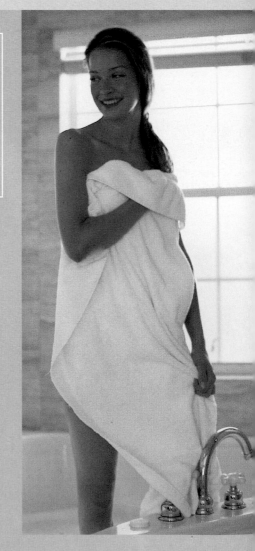

PLAN OF ACTION: 6 DAYS TO GO

- Every Morning routine (see page 84).
- Have your last facial and a body mask.
- Make final dress and hair adjustments if necessary after yesterday's dress rehearsals.
- Do final beauty checks and make any corrections and changes that you need to.
- Every Evening wind-down (see page 86).

---

last facial

Take time over your facial this evening. After cleansing and exfoliating, pour hot water on to half a lemon, some rose petals, a handful of lavender and camomile. Throw in some rosemary for oily skin or bay leaf for dry. Steam for 5 or 10 minutes and then splash with cool water.

Include a long, slow face massage, using the techniques presented on pages 74–75.

Indian bridal body mask

Mix 1 tablespoon each of powdered orange peel, powdered lemon peel and ground thyme with 2 tablespoons ground almonds, 4 tablespoons finely ground wheatgerm, half a teaspoon turmeric and a pinch of salt. Add enough almond oil to make a paste, and a few drops of rose or jasmine essential oil. Spread over the entire body and leave for up to 20 minutes. Massage well before showering off.

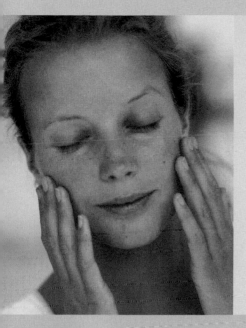

> **MENU: 6 DAYS TO GO**
>
> **Breakfast** Eggs on toast spread with yeast extract, a bowl of natural yogurt with honey, a glass of orange juice and ginger tea. Today's menu is the perfect pick-me-up if you're starting to feel run down after months of preparations or if you've been out for a drink the night before (in which case, add more fruit juice).
>
> **Lunch** Hummus sandwich with a watercress and tomato salad.
>
> **Dinner** Lamb chops or vegetarian grill served with brown rice, cabbage, red onions and chopped mint.
>
> **Snacks** Fruit salad of orange, kiwi fruit, strawberries and melon. An apple or pear.
>
> **Before bed** Toast and honey.
>
> **Drinks** Drink lots of water and fruit juice throughout the day.

Above Take time over your facial tonight. It's the last one you'll have before your wedding day, so make it a luxurious ritual. Bask in the fragrance of rose petals and the stimulating freshness of herbs.

Left After your facial and the rare luxury of a full-body bridal mask, take time for a relaxing bath before going to bed. Warm is better than hot, as it promotes restful sleep.

final beauty check & corrections

- Has your skin tone changed since your wedding make-up practice session? Even without a tan, your skin is likely to have a warmer colour in the summer, whereas winter skin is pale and cool. Check now to see whether you need to adjust your make-up.
- Has the shape of your face changed – for example, has weight loss made your cheekbones more visible? You may require subtly different contouring.
- Do you tend to blush or go pale with emotion? Use a little colour-corrective make-up or blusher. Also take into account your reaction to heat, if the venue full of friends and relatives is likely to be hot.
- If you're marrying in an exotic location, take account of the different climate and conditions.
- If you need to use camouflage make-up, for a scar or a tattoo, have you had a trial run?
- Has sunny weather left tan lines on your chest or shoulders? If you exfoliate thoroughly and stay covered up, they may fade before the wedding. Meanwhile, practise with foundation and powder.
- Are your nails in good shape to be shown off? If not, don't risk trying false nails now if you haven't tried them before. Just smooth off the nails, use lots of hand cream and paint them with clear polish instead of coloured.
- Is your hair the right length for the hairstyle you've chosen? If you need a trim, do it now so that it's settled down before the day. But if you were expecting it to have grown more than it has, now is the time to practise an alternative style.

5 days to go

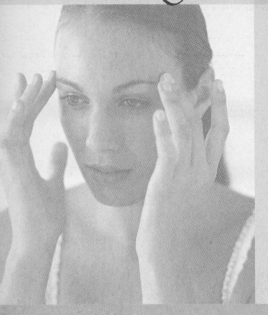

There are bound to be hiccups when planning a wedding and you might inadvertently be letting problems crease your brow. If you're not sure whether you are, put a bit of sticky tape between your eyebrows when no one's around. If you feel it crinkling, let a long breath out, and consciously release tension from your forehead.

When pressure builds up, relax your face with a 5-minute massage. You can use the European massage techniques below, or try the eastern tradition of acupressure opposite, which aims to increase 'vital energy' in the body.

PLAN OF ACTION: 5 DAYS TO GO
- Every Morning routine (see page 84).
- Do anything you still need to after yesterday's final beauty checks.
- Put sticky tape on your forehead to check whether you're frowning.
- Focus on releasing tension from your face.
- Give yourself a 5-minute facial massage.
- Every Evening wind-down (see page 86).

massage techniques

You can do without oil if you're mainly using static pressure, as in the facial massage opposite, or moving skin a small distance over underlying tissue, as in the hand and head and shoulder massages (see pages 98 and 100). To do **'thumb circles'**, for example, you press with the thumb pad and move the skin over the muscle or bone. This works well anywhere on your body, and it's an easy way to ease tension across your temples and around your jaw.

Work with the pads of your fingers – the soft part at the back of the top joint – rather than the fingertips, which are too sharp. For long, invigorating strokes, use **'piano-player fingers'**: extended and slightly curved, strong but without tension, as if about to play the piano. Use

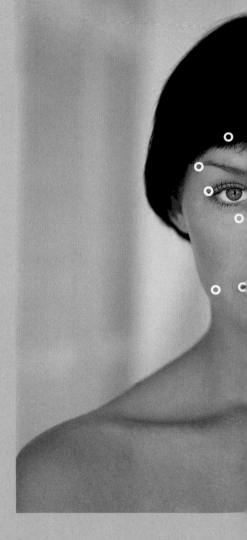

Right You may not have noticed tension building up, but it creates lines. To ease it, work gently on the acupressure points on your face.

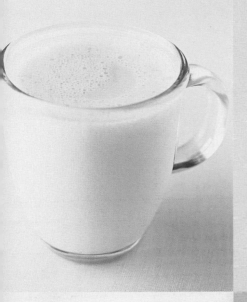

MENU: 5 DAYS TO GO

Breakfast Pumpkin Seed and Apricot Muesli (see page 70), a glass of unsweetened grapefruit juice.

Lunch A can of lentil soup, plus a slice of bread topped either with 75 g (3 oz) drained canned tuna in brine with a dash of lemon juice, or with hummus. Add sliced tomato and a handful of alfalfa sprouts.

Dinner Grilled 150 g (5 oz) chicken breast or vegetarian grill; with couscous and grilled vegetables such as red pepper and courgette.

Snacks Half a mango topped with low-fat cottage cheese. Two satsumas or kiwi fruit.

Before bed A glass of milk.

Drinks Drink plenty of water, and try peppermint tea if nerves are making your stomach churn.

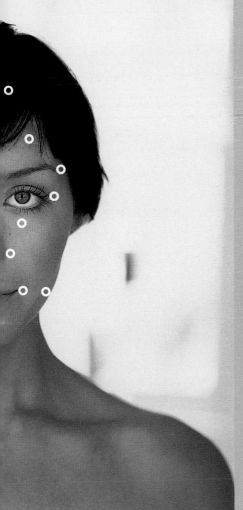

light pressure to stimulate circulation: deeper pressure, used to squeeze tension out of the long muscles, needs oil to prevent the skin dragging. A simple massage rule is always to put pressure on muscle, not on joints.

5-minute facial acupressure

Before you begin, wash your face and hands and take out contact lenses if you wear them. Sit in front of a mirror, but start with your eyes closed and try to feel small indentations at the points illustrated on the left. Keep your eyes shut and let your fingers explore until they slip into the spot. The acupressure points often feel like small hollows in the bone or at junctions, and may feel softer or stickier than the surrounding tissue. If you're not certain, check in the mirror.

1 **Warm up** Rub your hands together to warm them, then shake out any tension. Most of the main facial acupressure points shown are in pairs, so work on both at the same time.

2 **Exert some pressure** Press with the tips of your fingers, avoiding your nails, for up to 10 seconds at each point. Exert a light to medium pressure of about 1.5 kg (3¼ lb) – check on your kitchen scales as to how that feels. For a lighter touch, use your third fingers. Increase the pressure gradually at the beginning and ease off at the end.

3 **On-the-spot massage** Massage on the spot in tiny circular movements without stretching or pulling. The skin should move over the bone, not your fingers over the skin.

4 **Know when to stop** If it hurts, stop at once, but if you feel slight resistance or discomfort, continue. Repeat up to three times at each spot.

4 days to go

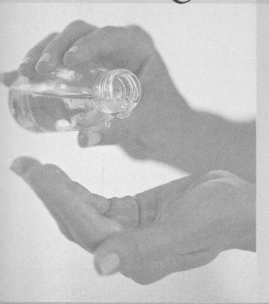

Make up an emergency repair kit in good time, and give it to your chief bridesmaid or other helper to carry for you. This should contain everything you might need on the day, such as oil blotting papers and powder in case your skin starts to shine, and baby wipes in case you need to clean your fingers. Small containers of your main items of make-up, such as foundation, will allow you to do running repairs without any drama. Put them in a purse small enough for her to carry in her own bag. Then turn your bathroom into a spa for the evening and relax.

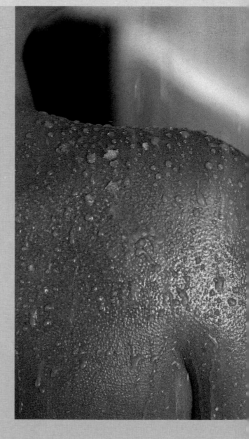

PLAN OF ACTION: 4 DAYS TO GO
- Every Morning routine (see page 84).
- Make up an emergency repair kit for your chief bridesmaid to carry on the day.
- Ensure that you have tried out everything in the kit.
- Make up some scented oil and prepare a scrub for your skin.
- Give yourself a home spa relaxing treatment.
- Every Evening wind-down (see page 86).

home spa

1 **Set the scene** Light a few candles, put on some soothing music and give notice that you're taking over the bathroom. Start by dry brushing your whole body (see page 72), then exfoliate with your favourite scrub, take a warm shower and rinse off well.

2 **Aromatherapy** Run a warm bath with your favourite aromatherapy oil. If you can bear the thought of a lukewarm bath, try running one that's just about body temperature: you can hardly tell, when you test it with your hand, whether your hand is in the water or not. This is the most refreshing temperature. A hot bath damages your skin and can stop you sleeping well.

3 **Have a good soak** Soak in the bath water for 10–20 minutes, with a glass of water or fruit juice with sparkling water on hand. If the bath's lukewarm, top it up every now and then with warm water. Finish with a cool shower if you wish, to invigorate your skin.

4 **Rub in oil** Massage scented almond oil (see box opposite) into your

Above Take a warm shower after dry brushing and exfoliating. Warm water is kinder to your skin than hot, and also helps you sleep better. Raising your temperature can keep you awake.

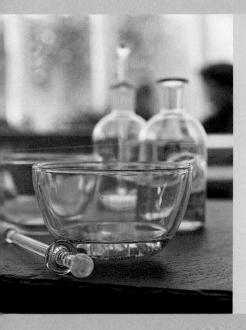

MENU: 4 DAYS TO GO

Breakfast Porridge with dried fruit and skimmed milk, and a cup of peppermint tea.

Lunch Salmon with a squeeze of lemon, or a vegetarian grill, served with a mixed green salad with artichoke hearts.

Dinner Quick Lentil Salad (see page 70), served with couscous or quinoa.

Snacks Natural yogurt with fruit salad. A handful of almonds, peanuts or sunflower seeds.

Before bed A slice of Granary, soya or barley bread with cottage cheese and lettuce.

Drinks Fruit juice mixed with water. Tap water is usually fine, but also try fizzy mineral water to add a sparkle.

Above Choose a base oil to suit your skin before adding your favourite essential oils. Almond and grapeseed are the classic bases; try sesame if your skin is dry, and jojoba or sunflower if it's oily or blemished.

whole body. If you don't like the feel of oil remaining on your skin, do this after the warm shower and before getting into the bath. Finally, go to bed and enjoy a blissfully long sleep.

emergency repair kit checklist

As with everything else you're using on the day, make sure you've tried all of the beauty products below in advance so as not to experience an adverse reaction. If you're decanting items such as foundation or mineral water into smaller containers, carry them around for a day beforehand to make sure they're watertight!

- Oil blotting papers and pressed powder to stop your skin shining
- Lipstick and lip salve, in case your mouth goes dry
- Tissues, to remove lipstick that needs reapplying
- Light-reflecting concealer
- Nail polish, to cover any chips
- A tiny container of foundation, to cover stray mascara if it smudges
- Cotton wool buds, to apply the foundation
- Make-up remover wipes
- White chalk (if your dress is white), to cover any marks
- A needle and white thread – just in case!
- Eye drops: simple saline for your eyes, strong vein-constrictor for red spots
- Painkillers, in case you get a headache
- Tampons, if required
- Peppermints, for your breath
- A mineral water facial spray for an instant lift

SCENTED MASSAGE OIL
To a tablespoon of almond oil, add two drops of one of the following essential oils:
- Rose or jasmine for dry skin
- Neem for damaged skin
- Lavender or tea tree for blemishes
- Lemon or bergamot for oily skin
- Lavender or geranium for normal skin

3 days to go

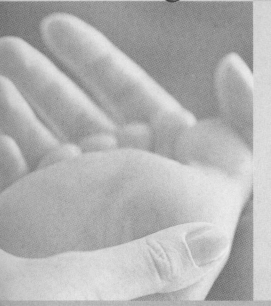

If you haven't already delegated tasks for the wedding day, now is the time to offload as much as possible on to reliable friends and relatives who are willing to help. Because the chief bridesmaid will be right behind you, she's the one who should carry a small bag of essentials for you, including your emergency repair kit (see page 95). If your bridesmaids aren't old enough to take responsibility, ask your mother or other reliable helper to look after it for you. When you have finished delegating, give yourself a full pedicure, including massage, and finish by painting your toenails.

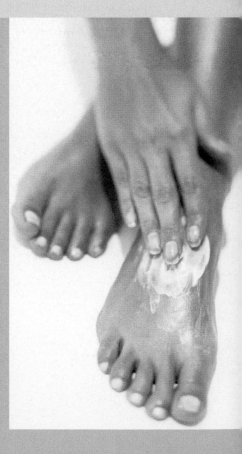

PLAN OF ACTION: 3 DAYS TO GO
- Every Morning routine (see page 84).
- Don't eat any salty food after today if it makes your eyes puffy.
- Delegate tasks for the wedding day to reliable helpers.
- Wax your legs and bikini line. If you're having this done professionally, get your eyebrows waxed into shape, too. Don't try this at home, unless you're very good at it.
- Have a full pedicure (see page 54) and foot massage, and paint your toenails.
- Slather your hands with nourishing cream or almond oil, and go to bed wearing cotton gloves.
- Every Evening wind-down (see page 86).

foot massage

Include this as part of your pedicure, sitting with your feet supported on a footstool. Use plenty of oil. Better still, get someone else to do it for you! Work gently on the foot, as there's very little flesh to cushion the delicate network of bones. But don't go so lightly that it tickles.

1 **Starting strokes** Start by stroking your foot from your toes to ankle. Knead the sole with your thumbs. Next, holding it in both hands, make large thumb circles over the whole of the top of your foot.

2 **Inside pressure** Grip the inside of your foot with your thumbs on the sole and pull your fingers and thumb gently towards each other. Most of the pressure is going from the thumb into the sole. If a helper is

Above Feet rarely get the kind of loving care they deserve. Start by washing them, drying carefully between the toes, then nurture them with plenty of oil or rich cream when you massage them.

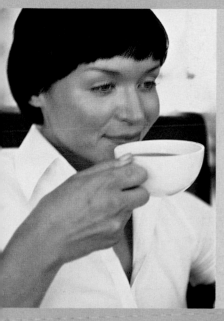

MENU: 3 DAYS TO GO

Breakfast A bowl of natural low-fat yogurt with apricots: fresh if in season, otherwise chopped dried apricots. A glass of carrot juice.
Lunch Omelette with optional diced ham, served with a green salad with avocado.
Dinner Baked potato with a tablespoonful of low-fat cottage cheese, baked beans and carrots, plus red onions sprayed with oil and grilled till they're tender.
Snacks Two oatcakes topped with cottage cheese and yeast extract. A handful of almonds.
Before bed A banana.
Drinks Drink water as usual, and try herbal teas such as camomile, to help you relax and sleep.

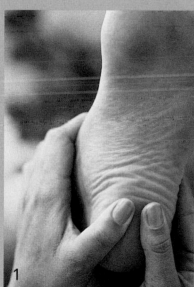

1

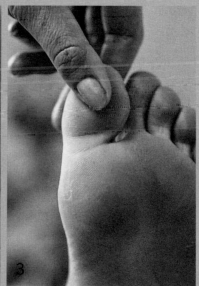

3

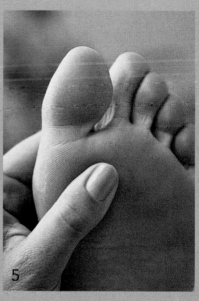

5

doing this for you, they can do the same on the outside of the foot.
3 **Individual treatment** Pull and knead each toe separately, then squeeze the pad of each toe and let go quickly.
4 **Knuckle down** Work on the sole of your foot with your knuckles. Then rub firmly with the thumb in a series of strokes from heel to toes, and make thumb circles all over the sole.
5 **Encourage relaxation** Work across the sole with thumb circles, just below the ball of the foot, and into the indentation in the centre.
6 **Finishing strokes** Finish by stroking firmly with piano-player fingers. Stroke briskly up the soles and top of the foot, over the ankle and towards the knee. Now repeat the massage on your other foot.

2 days to go

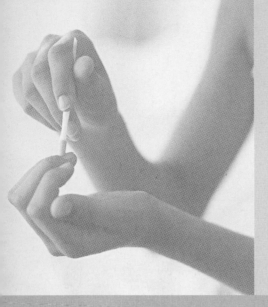

Give yourself plenty of time today for a slow, luxurious manicure, with relaxing music in the background. Include a hand massage: as with any massage, this will be all the better and more relaxing if someone else does it for you. Start your manicure by laying out everything you need, thinking of nothing except what you're doing. This is actually a meditation technique, known as 'mindfulness'. Enjoy the creativity of painting your nails, allowing plenty of time for each coat to dry. Try to keep this serenity, and the ability to focus on the present, throughout the coming days.

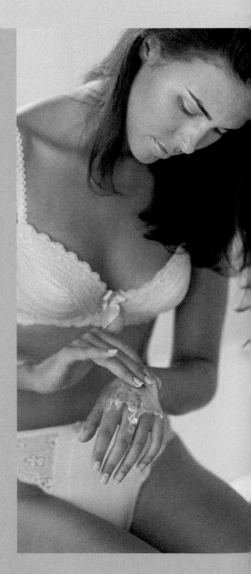

PLAN OF ACTION: 2 DAYS TO GO
- Every Morning routine (see page 84).
- Don't wear any make-up today – let your skin breathe.
- Put eyepads, or a bottle of rosewater, in the fridge ready for the wedding morning in case you forget tomorrow.
- Give yourself a manicure (see page 52) and hand massage and paint your nails.
- Every Evening wind-down (see page 86).

hand massage

1 **Warm up your hands** Prepare your favourite massage oil; plain almond is a traditional choice or use a stress-busting oil blend (see box opposite). Rub your hands together to warm them, then pour about a teaspoon of oil into your palms and work it into both hands as if 'washing' them. Cover the wrists, too, and work it well into and around the nails.

2 **Press the palm** Holding the left hand cupped in the right, gently press the palm with the pad of your right thumb. You can press quite firmly, but all your movements should be gentle and unhurried.

3 **Perform thumb circles** Massage with your thumb in small circular movements, not moving over the skin but moving the skin over the underlying tissue. Lift your thumb from the centre of the palm and repeat the massaging movement all over the palm.

4 **Massage your fingers** Hold your left fingers cupped in your right hand, and repeat the massaging movement, working up the fingers.

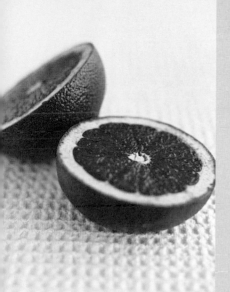

MENU: 2 DAYS TO GO
Breakfast Boiled egg with two rye crispbreads topped with yeast extract. Half a grapefruit, a smoothie made with 150 ml (1/4 pint) of skimmed milk and four handfuls of berries.
Lunch Bean salad: mix 50 g (2 oz) canned red kidney beans, at least 75 g (3 oz) cooked sliced green beans, 1/4 onion, finely chopped, 1 teaspoon chopped coriander, 1 teaspoon olive oil, and season to taste. Top with 100 g (31/2 oz) mackerel (optional), baby carrots and cherry tomatoes.
Dinner A 150-g (5-oz) salmon, Quorn™ or soya steak, served with asparagus spears, peas and new potatoes.
Snacks A slice of barley toast with peanut butter. An apple or orange.
Before bed A milky hot drink such as cocoa or a malt extract drink.
Drinks Drink plenty of water, preferably still spring water.

Left Hands harbour more tension than we realize, especially after weeks of writing lists and keeping notes on top of your normal work. Allow yourself to feel intuitively where you most need to massage.

Gently pull each finger and the thumb. (If you're feeling anxious, pinch one thumb while focusing on letting your breath out slowly several times.)

5 **Stroke in one direction** With brisker movements, extend the right-hand fingers as if about to play the piano, and stroke firmly down the front and back of the left hand towards the armpit, using your finger pads.

6 **Repeat and shake** Repeat the massage on the other hand. Finish by holding your hands away from your sides and shaking them vigorously.

head and hands

Relieve pre-wedding stress headaches. Starting from your wrist below the little finger, run the opposite index finger up and down the sides of your fingers and thumb as if drawing an outline of the hand. Do this slowly and mindfully, and repeat on the other hand.

STRESS-BUSTING OIL BLEND
Use the following blend of oils for a blissful body massage, or put it in an oil-burner to scent the room:

2 drops lavender essential oil
2 drops mandarin essential oil
1 drop jasmine essential oil
2 teaspoons grapeseed or almond oil

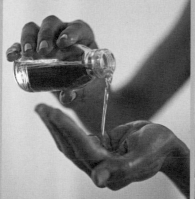

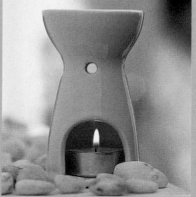

1 day to go

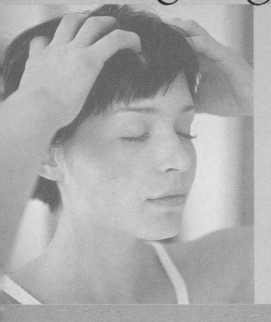

Try not to leave yourself with anything major to do today. The few last-minute beauty steps will be enough, along with a head and shoulder massage to help you relax before an early night. Spend some quiet time with your fiancé, enjoying each other's company. If any last-minute hitches or queries have cropped up, check that they're all resolved and you both know exactly what to do the next day. Remember, after all these months of planning, that the wedding is just one day – what it's really about is the future you're looking forward to together.

PLAN OF ACTION: 1 DAY TO GO
- Every Morning routine (see page 84).
- Wash your hair today instead of tomorrow, to help it hold its style.
- Exfoliate your lips by gently brushing with your toothbrush. Rehydrate with lip moisturizer or salve.
- Tidy your eyebrows. Don't make them thin (this can look harsh) or pluck away from the inner end. Just remove any stray hairs.
- Leave make-up off again today.
- If your dress reveals your shoulders and they are often marked by your bra straps, don't wear a bra today.
- Enjoy a head and shoulder massage to help you relax.
- Every Evening wind-down (see page 86).

head and shoulder massage

1 **Sit quietly and relax** Let your head fall forwards, and slowly swing it up to first one side and back and then the other. Raising your head again, lift and drop your shoulders. Squeeze and rub your upper arms.
2 **Massage the front of your shoulders** Using the knuckles of both hands pointing inwards, make circular kneading movements over the front of your shoulders, your upper arms and the back of your shoulders.
3 **Reach down your back** Using the pads of your fingers, press into the muscles beside the spine, as far down your back as you can reach. Make small, firm circular movements without moving your fingers over the skin. Lift them and repeat a finger's width higher up. Repeat until you've worked your way up to the top of the neck.

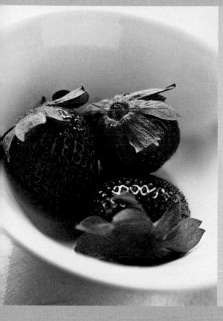

MENU: THE DAY BEFORE YOUR WEDDING

Breakfast Cereal with skimmed milk and berries, two slices of Granary or barley toast with mashed banana, a glass of orange juice.

Lunch Grilled chicken breast or tofu (bean curd), served with a salad of baby spinach leaves, red peppers, artichoke hearts and red cabbage.

Dinner Wholemeal spaghetti bolognese made with lean or vegetarian mince, tomatoes, peppers and aubergine, topped with two tablespoons of grated cheese.

Snacks Fruits rich in vitamin C, such as mango, guava, kiwi fruit, citrus fruit, strawberries or any kind of berries.

Before bed A banana smoothie made with soya or skimmed milk.

Drinks Drink as much water as you can throughout the day ready for the celebrations tomorrow.

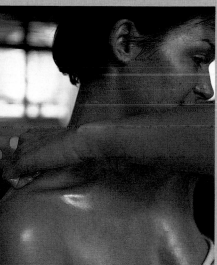

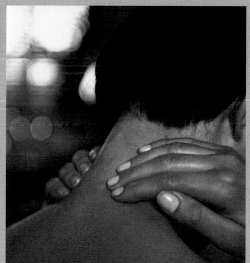

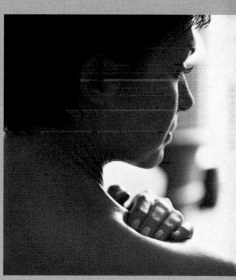

Above Knotted muscles can give you hunched shoulders and put a frown on your face. Knead the tension out of these long-suffering muscles with a massage that you can do with or without oil.

4 **Work the top of your shoulders** Working with one hand at a time on the opposite shoulder, apply slow, deep pressure to the muscle on top. Start at the outer end. Work your way along by lifting your fingers and repeating the pressure a finger's width nearer the neck.

5 **Do thumb circles** Cupping your hands over your head, spread your fingers out over the scalp and massage along under the edge of the skull from beside the ears towards the spine with thumb circles.

6 **Massage your scalp** With hands pressed firmly on each side of your head, push them towards each other, moving the scalp over the skull. Don't let your fingers slip across the scalp and pull your hair. With piano-player fingers, massage your scalp in small circles. Finish by running your fingers through your hair several times.

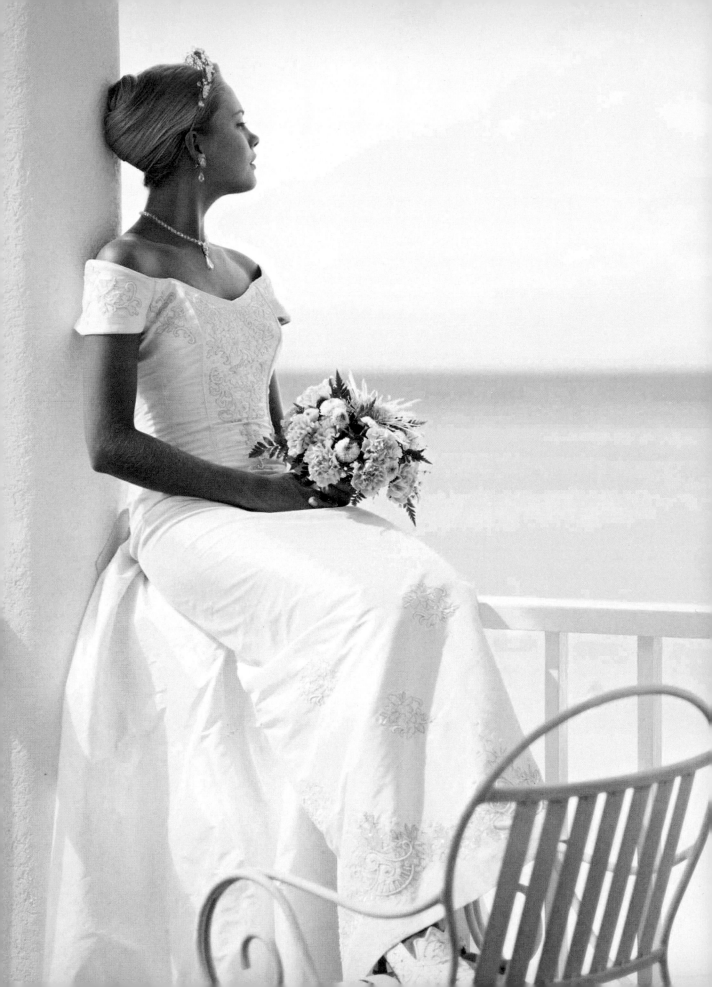

your wedding day

At last it's the day you've spent so much time preparing for. Set your alarm early, so you won't have to rush. Take a few quiet moments to visualize the day's events, all running smoothly. Picture the happiness on the faces of your family and friends.

Do some slow stretches, then have breakfast: a glass of fruit juice and a bowl of yogurt or non-sugary cereal, with a sliced banana to add some calming potassium. Then brush your skin and have a leisurely shower, remembering not to wash your hair today.

Try not to worry about details. Enjoy this unique day for everything it has to offer, taking time to notice all that's happening and fix it in your mind. People will barely notice, much less remember, whether the place cards perfectly matched the candles. What will stay with you and everyone else is whether you are radiating happiness or tension. If you do feel nervous, try the celebrities' stress-busting trick and smile – it works!

WEDDING PLANNING CHECKLIST: WEDDING DAY (AND AFTER)

Make sure your most reliable friend has organized who is going to:

- Check that the best man has the rings.
- Send your luggage to the first-night hotel.
- Take home your dress and the groom's suit if you change into going-away clothes.

- Pack and take home wedding presents, keeping note of who gave them.
- Return any hired items.
- Send out wedding cake to anyone who couldn't come on the day.

a stress-free start

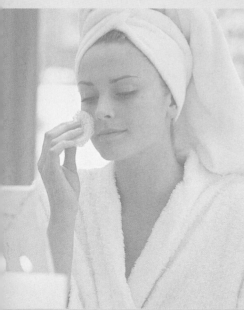

Have your clothes, including underwear, ready to put on, so you don't have to rummage for anything when you're coiffed and made up. Don't put on a bra that will leave marks if you're not going to wear it under your dress and, for the same reason, don't wear glasses if you're not intending to wear them later. Stay in your dressing-gown or wear a button-up shirt, that won't have to come off over your head.

Arrange well in advance with a reliable friend or relative to take charge of everything else that needs to be done this morning, so you have no distractions.

helping hands

A massage would be a soothing start to the morning's preparations. Use some of the oil-free techniques from pages 92–101, as a trace of oil could mark your dress. Or get someone to give you a luxurious full massage using a stress-busting oil blend (see page 99). You can always shower the oil off afterwards.

doing your hair

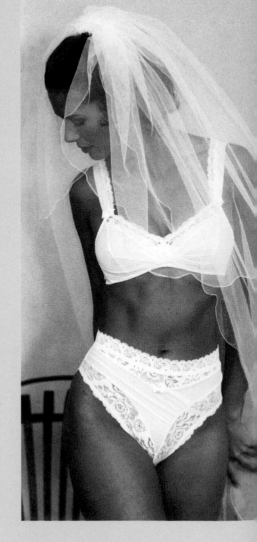

Put all your hair and make-up requirements on a table near a good light source, with at least one hand mirror and preferably a magnifying mirror. Pour a cup of camomile tea, pull up a comfortable chair and put a 'Do not disturb' sign on the door – for everyone who's not actively helping you get ready. Leave someone else in charge outside.

You'll probably be using more hair products than usual to hold the style, as long as you've had a successful trial run. But don't overload your hair, in case it collapses under the weight before the day is out.

Wearing a head-dress If your hair needs to be arranged around the head-dress, put it on now. If only minor adjustments will be needed – or if you need to put your dress on over your head – you can wait till after you've done your make-up and dressed. But don't leave it much later than that. If you're worried your head-dress will come loose, you need to make sure it's securely anchored. Concerns about your head-dress shouldn't restrict your movement: fix it now or you'll be worrying that it will fall off when you kiss your new husband.

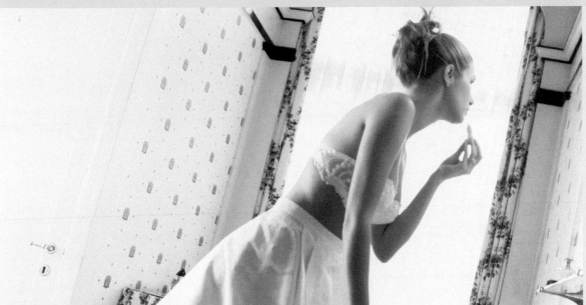

Above Find a quiet spot with good lighting, mirrors and space for all your hair and make-up products. Close the door and put up a 'do not disturb' sign for anyone except your designated helpers.

Left Putting your head-dress on as soon as your hair is ready gives you time to ensure that it's firmly fixed and won't slip. Then take off the veil till just before you leave.

take a break

When your hair is ready, cleanse your skin of any stray hair products.

If there's still plenty of time before the ceremony, pause for a break. You don't want to put your make-up on too soon – especially if you have oily skin – or it will be flagging by the time you're posing for photos after the wedding.

Have a snack of fruit and a wholemeal cheese and lettuce sandwich. If you're hungry enough, eat a simple meal of meat or tofu (bean curd) with vegetables or salad. It's a long time till the reception. You'll know best whether you're at risk of feeling sick if you eat, or fainting (or hearing your tummy rumble) if you don't.

emergency action

- **Got a spot?** Don't panic. If it's squeezable, this is the one time it's all right to squeeze – it can come back with a vengeance tomorrow. Otherwise, dab it with astringent, or the scent you're wearing (not with antiseptic because of the smell). Then pat it with concealer and powder over it.
- **Cold sore starting?** If you haven't got any antiviral cream, slap a cool used teabag on the spot.
- **Stomach churning?** Suck peppermints, nibble crystallized ginger, drink peppermint or ginger tea.
- **Puffy eyes?** Put a couple of spoons in the freezer, then lie down for a few minutes with the cold spoons cupping your eyes. Or use eyepads soaked in plain water or rosewater, kept in the fridge overnight.

TOP TIP
Once your hair has been styled, touch it as little as possible so it stays in shape.

getting dressed

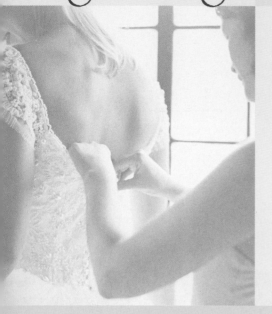

Start these final preparations in plenty of time before you have to leave the house. You don't want any last-minute hitches to make you chew your immaculate nail polish. Have one or two sensible, practical friends or relatives to run any last-minute errands that crop up. They should also help you to dress, as it's hard to do alone and you'd risk smearing your make-up. This can be a happy moment to share with your Mum, best friend or sisters. Just make sure in advance that they know what to do – and don't let a crowd of well-wishers get under your feet.

order of the day

Make-up Still in your dressing-gown, put on your make-up. Do this with the help of a friend if you've already practised this together. If it's being professionally done, you'll appreciate the make-up artist coming to you. You have enough to do without worrying about being held up or caught in a downpour on the way home from your visit.

Lingerie Next, put on your bridal lingerie. Take enough time to check that everything is straight and doesn't slip out of place when you sit or move around.

The dress Get someone to undo all the fastenings and put the dress on the floor where you can step carefully into it in bare feet, holding something steady for support. Stay upright while your helpers lift the dress for you to slip your arms in, and do it up for you.

If the opening on your dress isn't wide enough to step into, you'll need to have it put on over your head. In this case, drape a thin scarf over your face and hair. Raise your arms above your head. Get two agile helpers to stand on chairs beside you and lift the dress so it drops down neatly without rumpling your hair or smearing your make-up. If your skirt has a bustle or train, let your helpers arrange these.

Your shoes Have your shoes set out ready for you to step straight into. Carefully lift your skirt away from your feet as you take a few steps to get used to the feeling, although you should have already practised walking in the dress and shoes.

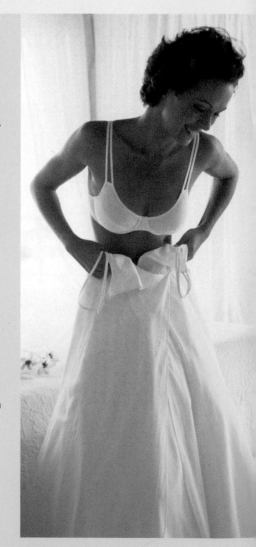

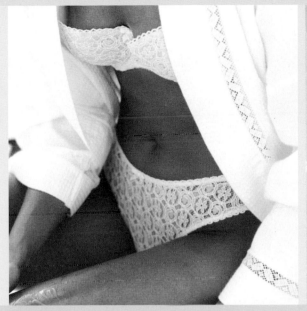

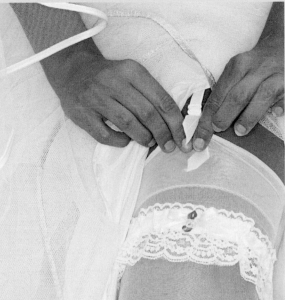

Above This is one day when white or nude are the only colour options for underwear, if you're wearing a white dress. Any other colours might show through. And when else would you wear a garter?

Left A slip is a vital foundation for certain styles of wedding dress, ensuring that your silhouette remains smooth and the dress hangs and moves perfectly.

Final touches Practise moving with a bustle or train. Practise sitting down, puffing the skirt out around you if it is full, or discreetly lifting it a little at the hips to make room if it is tightly fitted. Gather the skirt carefully in one hand as you walk up and down the stairs, keeping it clear of your feet without crushing the fabric. If you're wearing a veil, put it on and arrange it now.

Leaving the house If you're travelling to the wedding venue by car or other transport, allow for your head-dress and lift your skirt away from your feet as you step into the car. Pull your skirt up at the back while you're in the vehicle, and lean forward to avoid wrinkling it. Step out carefully, holding your skirt clear of the ground. Relax, take a deep breath, walk into your future, and have a wonderful time.

RUNNING REPAIRS DURING THE DAY

Eyes If you smudge your mascara, dip a cotton wool bud in foundation and cover it up.

Lips Take lipstick off and reapply, rather than topping it up, so that the colour remains even. Wipe off the old lipstick with a tissue, stroking towards the inside of your mouth to avoid smearing it on to your face.

Face Keep a spray bottle handy, filled with plain water from the fridge: anything else might stain your dress when you give yourself a cooling spritz. Make sure it's got a safe top.

Hair A can of medium-hold hairspray will help keep your style in place. You may need Mum and her large handbag to hold this and your make-up kit.

photo-fit

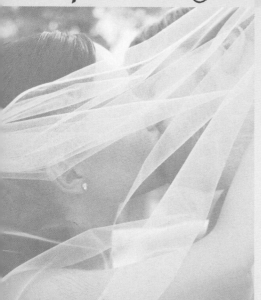

Your friends and family will think you look lovely. Ensure that the evidence backs them up by looking radiant in the photos. If you haven't shaped up or improved your skin as much as you'd hoped, this is your chance to use all the tricks of the trade to your advantage.

First, choose the right photographer and videographer. Before hiring a professional, visit studios to see if you like their wedding work. If you'd like some informal shots for your album, invite a friend to record preparations and other behind-the-scenes moments too.

all right in black and white

If you're having your photos and video taken by friends, try to have a dry run beforehand. You'll get an idea of what works and what angles suit you. See pages 78–81 for wedding make-up tips.

Black-and-white photographs add an artistic touch, and Victorian-style sepia photographs make an unusual keepsake. But different make-up rules apply, so it may be worth dressing up again and having these taken afterwards. A good coverage of foundation makes a flawless base for these photos. Don't be afraid to use enough blusher to create contours, but blend everything carefully, as demarcation lines will be visible. Strong eye and lip colours make a dramatic effect, but remember that reds appear black in non-colour photographs, and can make all but the most luscious lips look thin. Similarly, dark eye shadow can make your eyes look smaller.

the right angle

Look closely to see whether you photograph better from one side or another, and in full-face or profile. In close-ups, try turning your shoulders to about 45 degrees from the camera and looking back towards the camera, but still not quite full-face on. This popular angle flatters most faces and makes you look slimmer.

For full-length photos, stand at an angle to the camera, pushing your hips forwards and your shoulders back. With your back foot parallel to your body, point your front foot towards the camera, then turn to look at the camera.

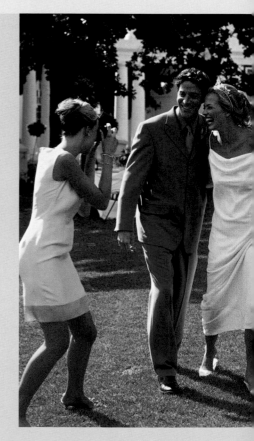

Above Informal photos by guests are often your best souvenirs. Let keen snappers know in advance if you'd welcome copies of their photos. Hand out and collect disposable cameras on the day.

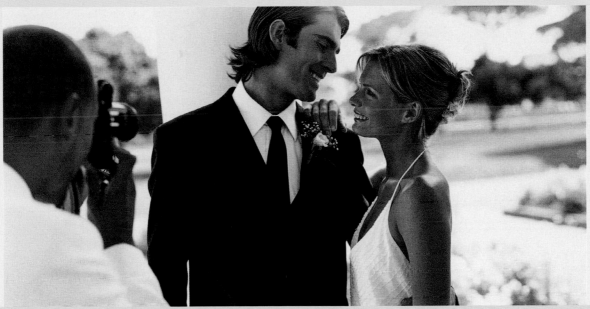

Above Flawlessly made-up, relaxed and happy, you'll reap the benefits of your preparations – both on the day and when you and your bridegroom look through the album of photographs.

the right place

Outdoor light is fine for large family groups, but for close-ups it may make you look washed out. Bright sunshine can cast unattractive shadows, and shows up signs of age or tiredness. If the light is coming from behind you, not shining on you, your face will be too indistinct.

Soft but solid (not dappled) shade is most flattering. Dark-skinned brides will want to be photographed against a fairly dark background, to prevent contrast problems.

Warm indoor light can work well, too – check out the venue in advance, at the time of day you'll be there. Non-professionals tend to use a simple flash for indoor photos. This washes out fair skin, but it may benefit dark-skinned brides (if they've used enough powder to prevent shine) by showing their features more clearly than in an amateur shot without a flash. Remind everyone to use red-eye reduction: the camera will flash several times.

If you prefer a sunny spot, turn your head away, then look back just before the click, so you're not squinting.

Don't be too serious about where and when you're photographed. Your album, and wedding-present frames, just need a few gorgeous pictures in the right conditions. Snaps by family and friends may turn out to be your most cherished souvenirs.

the ultimate cheat

If the worst happens (which it hardly ever does), you can always have more photos taken later. You would not be the first bride to do this!

TOP TIP
If you have the slightest hint of a double chin, make sure all photos are taken from your face level or higher. If the photographer's kneeling down, your throat will look its worst, showing up signs of age, extra weight or gauntness caused by crash dieting. If you can't escape pictures being taken from that unflattering angle, just bury your nose in your bouquet!

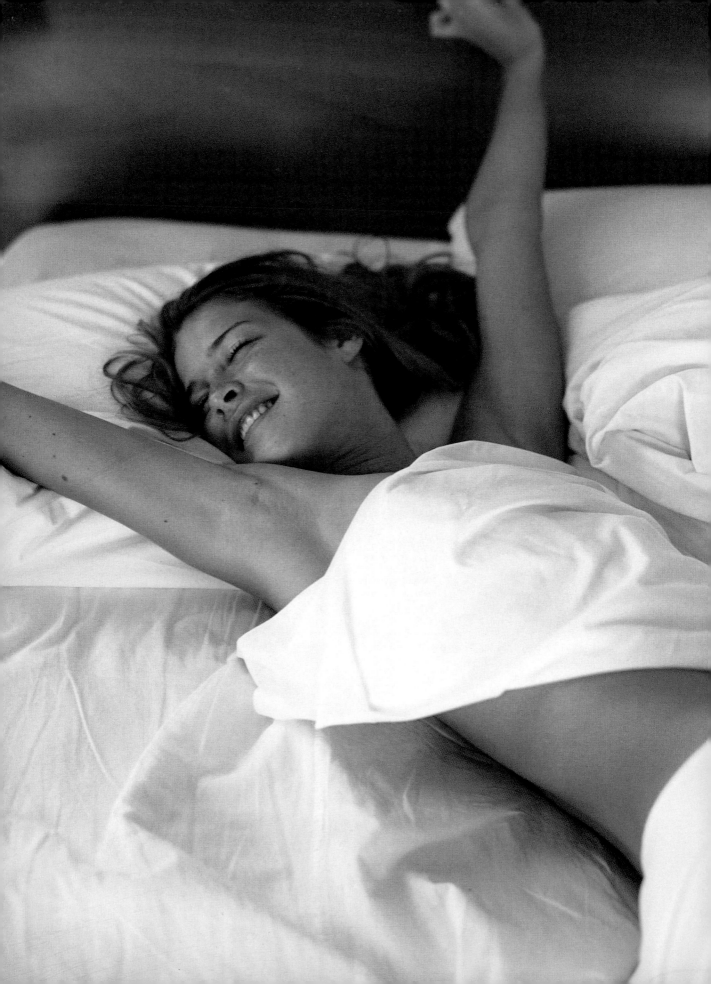

6-week fit bride plan

Six weeks to go and you've been too busy organising the wedding to think of yourself? Or have all the celebrations left you straining the seams of your dress?

Whatever the reason for your tight schedule, if you're serious about shaping up for your wedding, there's still time to make a noticeable difference. A targeted workout routine will help you shape up the parts that matter most in a wedding dress: your arms, bust and waist. Following the stringent but very healthy eating plan you can lose extra weight safely without wrecking your skin. Instead, you'll create a peachy complexion, with smooth skin and masses of energy to enjoy the day.

A few useful tricks will make you look taller and slimmer than you really are. Learning to walk elegantly in a long dress will repay the short time it takes. Even standing the right way can make the difference between an average picture and a photographic triumph.

6-week beauty plan

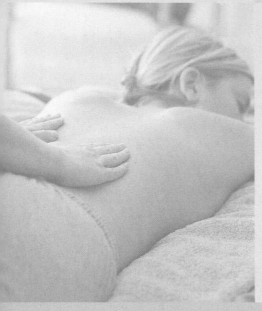

Planning is essential. Circle everything in the 6-week list on these pages that needs to be booked: hairdresser, salon treatments and so on. Make all these appointments during the first week, then phone two days before each one to reconfirm.

Keep a notebook for your plans and to-do lists, with a pen and a highlighter, so you're never searching for the scrap of paper on which you jotted a vital number. At home, keep everything relating to the wedding in a box file: useful now, and a treasured souvenir afterwards.

week 1

- During the first week of the 6-week Fit Bride Plan, you'll be detoxing with a juice fast and special exercises (see pages 114–116).
- Ask your hairdresser for advice on styles and head-dresses. Any big changes such as a perm or colour should be done now to give them time to settle. Have a trim and conditioning treatment now.
- Start weekly facials and exfoliation.
- If you're planning a series of salon treatments, check when they need to start and finish. Don't start any major treatments such as skin peels – there's not enough time to recover.
- Have a dental check-up and tooth polishing. If you're planning to have your teeth whitened, do it now.

week 2

- Start a focused exercise and eating plan (see pages 118–121).
- Begin fat-burning and body-sculpting exercises (see pages 122–125).
- It's worth investing in at least one professional treatment such as a facial. Get all the advice you can and write it down.
- Have your eyebrows shaped, then keep them in the same shape. If doing it yourself, avoid plucking them too thin or too far apart.
- Ask your best friend to come with you to all treatments and take digital or Polaroid photos. Use these to adapt and correct your look till you're satisfied.
- Start daily facial massage.
- Delegate everything possible to a reliable friend – or your mother.

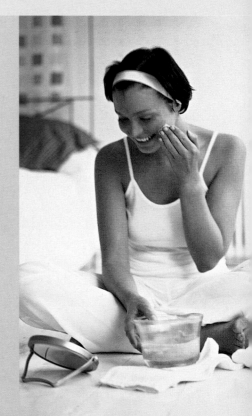

Above Start having regular facials as soon as possible, using gentle products or recipes that show their benefits at once, and discarding any that upset your skin. Don't try anything drastic such as a peel.

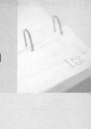

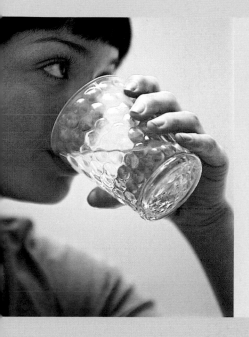

Above Drink more water than usual over the next six weeks. You'll be cutting down on other drinks, so you don't want to risk running low on fluids. And water should give your skin an extra sparkle.

week 3

- If you've previously had any problems triggered by stress, such as acne or eczema, see your doctor now. You may be recommended a preventive treatment.
- Consider taking a lesson from a make-up artist – cosmetic counters in department stores may offer a free session. Wear a top in the same shade as your dress and get a friend to take photos. Take notes and buy any products you want to use.
- If you're planning to use fake tan, try it now at the latest.
- Start using intensive creams on your hands and feet every day.

week 4

- Even if someone else is doing your hair on the day, have a trial run with your hairdresser to find a style that works. Wear a top with a similar neckline to your dress and get a friend to take photos.
- Use your last face mask before the day, in case it brings up spots.
- Learn the massage techniques shown on pages 92–101 with your fiancé, and massage each other whenever you need it.

week 5

- Aim to have everything ready by now if possible, to avoid stress in the final few days.
- Make final alterations to the dress.
- Do a final make-up rehearsal. Check that you have all the products you're going to use.

week 6

- Hold your hen night the first day of this week at the latest if you're planning a wild party. Otherwise, boost your shaping-up efforts with a group afternoon at a spa or beauty salon – a celebration that would leave you all looking good in the wedding photos.
- Try not to have any treatments, other than for relaxation, scheduled this week. Don't do or use anything new, in case of skin reactions.
- Follow instructions for the final week and wedding day from pages 82–109, with one exception. If you're feeling energetic enough, continue the full workout programme up till three days before the wedding. Then ease down with one rest day, one day of the Sunday routine (including a 40-minute exercise session) from pages 84–85 and a final day of rest.

week 1: detox

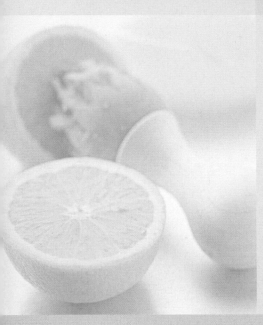

A stringent healthy eating plan can help you shed extra weight, give you the best complexion you've ever had and boost your energy levels significantly.

Don't go on a crash diet, though. You'd end up looking and feeling terrible on the day – and on your honeymoon. If you really can't squeeze into your wedding dress, it's better to relax and have it altered.

Follow this mild detoxifying regime for the first week to give yourself a flying start in shedding excess weight, relieving any puffiness and clearing your skin.

detoxing

The standard western diet contains a lot of chemical residues and saturated fat. Processed food is also full of sugar and artificial sweeteners and low in natural fibre, leaving many people slightly constipated. All this is bad news for your skin and waistline. A mild detox diet helps you break harmful habits and gives your body a chance to cleanse itself.

Stock up with fresh organic fruit and vegetables, and buy or borrow a juicer (see page 66 for recipes). If this is impossible, use a variety of the best-available, bought vegetable juices.

Don't go on a water-only fast – you burn muscle long before you start burning fat.

emotional release

Detoxing can take a lot out of you in more ways than one, so try not to be too active this week. You may get sugar and caffeine withdrawal symptoms for the first few days, and many people have unexpected emotional reactions. Your physical energy levels may drop as you become inward-looking – use the time for reflection and meditation. You'll be more than repaid with the energy you'll feel afterwards.

drinks

While you're detoxing, drink your fill of juice at mealtimes. Through the day, drink as much water as you like, either hot or at room temperature.

VEGETABLE BROTH

This traditional cleansing recipe, rich in minerals and antioxidants, features in the 1-week Detox and aims to counteract the acidic effects of our everyday diet. In addition, celery is a diuretic and will reduce bloating caused by water retention.

Take about two average-sized organic potatoes, carrots, celery sticks and beetroot. Scrub well and slice into a saucepan containing at least 1 litre (1 3/4 pints) of water. Bring to the boil, cover and cook over a low heat for at least 1 hour, adding more water if more than half has evaporated.

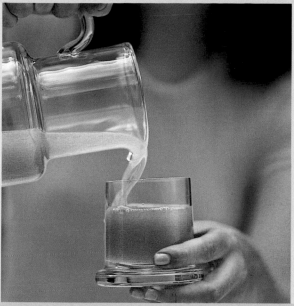

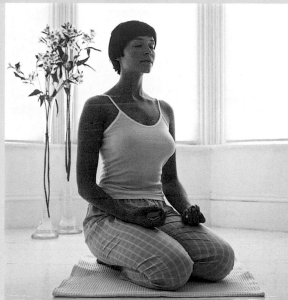

Above Fruit juices make a healthy and delicious detox breakfast, but contain too much natural sugar to drink all day. For lunch and dinner, try to have at least three different fresh vegetable juices.

Above right The detox process can make you feel less active and more reflective. Go along with this: give yourself time to meditate and to be alone with your thoughts.

1–week detox

Days 1 and 2
Breakfast A bowl of fresh fruit with natural low-fat yogurt. Omit the yogurt on Day 2.
Lunch and tea Steamed vegetables and salad. Season with any herbs you like, and dress the salad with herbs and lemon juice.
Dinner Vegetable broth (see box opposite).
Snacks Fresh vegetable sticks.

Day 3
Breakfast Fresh fruit juices.
Lunch, tea and dinner Fresh juices, mainly vegetable.

Day 4
Breakfast Fresh fruit juices.
Lunch and tea Fresh juices, mainly vegetable.
Dinner Vegetable broth (see box opposite).

Day 5
As for Day 1, but without the yogurt at breakfast.

Day 6
As for Day 1, but have the yogurt at lunchtime instead of breakfast.

Day 7
As for Day 1, but add tofu (bean curd), nuts and seeds at lunch.

week 1: look tall and light

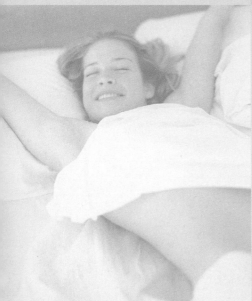

Start your 6-week fitness plan with gentle but powerful exercises that prepare your body for the work to come. This is the time to create the illusion of height and lightness, so that you'll walk down the aisle with dancer-like grace. A posture and stretch routine will lengthen and loosen your muscles. You'll also be doing exercises to boost the flow of lymph, aiding the body's cleansing process and giving you flawless skin.

You can adapt this timetable to suit your working hours, but start each morning with the exercises.

detox workout routine

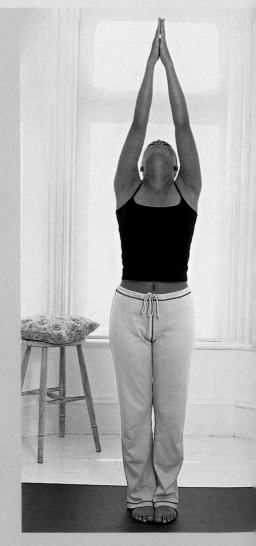

7am: wake up
- Spend a few minutes visualizing the day ahead in a positive way. Anticipate the pleasure of a relaxing beauty treatment, the sense of achievement as you tick another task off your 'to do' list. If any worries come up, put them on a 'to do' list and don't give them any further thought till after breakfast.
- Drink some warm water or peppermint tea.
- Do some breathing exercises (see page 60) – now and whenever you feel stressed throughout the day.

7.10am: detox exercise routine
- Start by linking your hands above your head and stretching upwards, feeling the stretch throughout your entire body.
- Having woken up your muscles, do the Standing Tall exercise on page 65, in front of a mirror. Take a few moments to correct your posture and try to re-establish this throughout the day.
- Now do some stretches from page 11.
- Continue with the lymph-boosting routine, pages 62–63.

7.30am: brush up
- Brush your skin all over (see page 72) to help boost lymph circulation, carrying out of your body the waste matter that dulls your skin.
- Take a warm shower, ending with a blast of cold. Try to stay under the cold water for at least a minute. Imagine you're enjoying a refreshing downpour in a tropical rainforest!

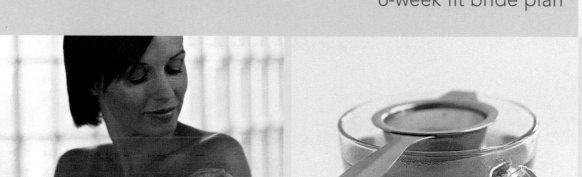

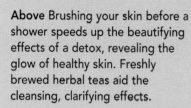

Above Brushing your skin before a shower speeds up the beautifying effects of a detox, revealing the glow of healthy skin. Freshly brewed herbal teas aid the cleansing, clarifying effects.

Left Start the day with a long, slow stretch to the sky, keeping your shoulders relaxed and neck long as you glance upwards. Continue the stretch while looking ahead.

During the day
Take any opportunity throughout the day to do some stretches and the toning exercises on pages 18–19.

Walk like a queen
Practise for your walk down the aisle. Starting with the Standing Tall exercise (see page 65), imagine you are a doll suspended from the ceiling by a string attached to the crown of your head. This image holds your head high, but without your jaw jutting upwards, crushing the back of your neck. Your neck lengthens as your shoulders relax. Step out at a relaxed pace, putting the ball of your foot down first, keeping your pelvis level and your head – not your chin – high.

6.30pm: wind down
Mark the transition from the working day to your own time when you arrive home by meditating for 10 minutes (see page 86). Use this as an opportunity to clear your mind. This actually helps you focus better the rest of the time on the things you have to do.

6.40pm: work out
On alternate evenings, perform:
1 The warm-up routine on page 10; or
2 The aerobic dance routine on pages 12–13, without music and at a gentle 'walk-through' pace.

Before bed
Give your face some gentle manual lymphatic drainage (see page 74).

weeks 2-6: superfast diet

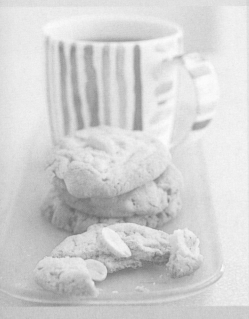

One week into the 6-week Fit Bride Plan and you've hit the ground running. Now you're going to cut out sugar and processed food. It sounds drastic, but few things have such a quick and visible effect on your skin and your body shape. You've already survived a week without them. Any withdrawal symptoms should already be past. You'll find that switching to a healthier diet gives you more energy. This will allow you to prepare real foods and still have time left over, and the benefits to your skin and shape will motivate you. See pages 22–25 and 44–49 for more healthy eating ideas.

the truth about sugar addiction

Sugar addiction is a bit of a myth. In reality, you're in control. Simply decide not to eat sugar or junk foods for the next five weeks, and get on with your life. If you do get an attack of the munchies:

● Ask yourself whether you're really desperate for sugar? Or are you tired, stressed, bored, thirsty or depressed? Stop and think what you really want – often it's something other than food. Then give yourself what you need.

● Procrastinate. Promise yourself a doughnut if that's what you really want, but in 10 minutes. By then the urge may have worn off.

● Do some exercise. It takes your mind off food and reminds you why you want to get fit.

● Have a sniff of vanilla – this has been proven to reduce sugar cravings. Just don't use vanilla ice cream!

WHY CUT OUT SUGAR AND PROCESSED FOOD?

Sugar isn't especially harmful in itself, but we eat unhealthy amounts of it. Because it's cheap and tasty, it's used in most processed food, even savouries. Junk foods – highly processed fast food, snacks and convenience meals – are also heavy in fat, of the cheapest and unhealthiest sort.

give yourself time

If this way of eating is a major change for you, it might take a while for your body to adjust. Eating more fruit and vegetables will give your bowel a lot more work, disconcerting if you're used to the constipating effects of a diet high in processed foods. It's not unhealthy to have two or three bowel movements a day. As long as it's not unstoppable and sudden, it's not diarrhoea – just your body adjusting to a better diet.

Check with your doctor before starting exercise or making any major changes. If you're on a special diet for health reasons, don't change it without medical advice.

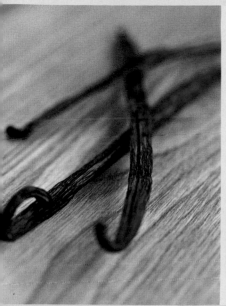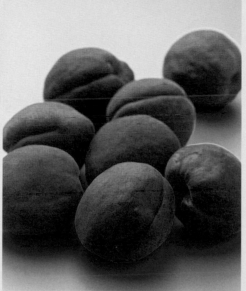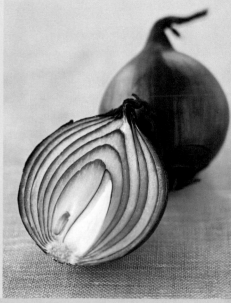

the superfast pyramid

This pyramid shows what to eat each day. See page 21 for explanations of serving sizes. Weigh all your food for the first week, to see whether you need to cut down portion sizes. Remember you can always fill up with non-starchy vegetables. The pyramid gives you the basic rules, while the meal ideas overleaf show you just how easy they are to follow

Above Soothe your sweet tooth the natural way, with a sniff of vanilla pod, the juiciness of ripe apricots or the surprising rich sweetness of cooked red onions.

Nuts, seeds, legumes and their oils: one serving a day.

Dairy foods such as yogurt and cheese, preferably low-fat: one or two servings a day.

Meat, fish, eggs and other high-protein foods: one to three servings a day, including oily fish at least three times a week.

Starchy foods (wholemeal bread, wholegrain cereals, rice): two to three servings a day.

Fruit: three to four servings a day.

Vegetables: at least six servings a day of any vegetables and salads. Not more than one-third of these should be root vegetables such as potatoes and parsnips.

weeks 2-6: curb the cravings

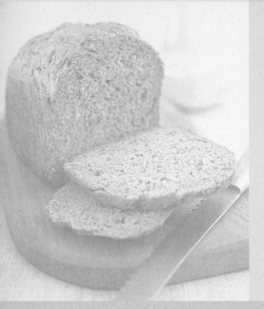

These meal ideas contain plenty of nutrients that stop you feeling hungry. Eat three satisfying meals a day, with an optional two snacks. Add as many vegetables and salads as you like. Don't skip any meals, and don't replace more than one solid meal a day with juices. If you overeat one day, don't try to compensate the next – just return to the recommended pattern. Drink plenty of hot or cold water, and beware of diet foods. 'Low-fat' products usually contain extra sugar, while 'reduced-sugar' foods often contain artificial sweeteners, which may increase your cravings.

breakfast

Choose one of the following, plus herbal tea or fruit juice:
- Sugar-free cereal with a sprinkling of wheatgerm, fresh chopped fruit and milk.
- A handful of dried apricots, cranberries and apples soaked in water, topped with natural yogurt.
- Toast with yeast extract instead of butter.
- Grilled bacon, mushrooms (sprayed with a mist of oil) and tomatoes.
- Scrambled egg with pepper and thyme. Toast with yeast extract instead of butter.
- Porridge made with water, topped with a handful of raisins.
- Prunes in juice with low-fat fromage frais.

lunch

Have one of the options below, with one or two pieces of fruit:
- A wholemeal yeast-extract sandwich with piles of salad leaves.
- Organic ham with a large mixed salad, including alfalfa sprouts.
- Apples, a hard-boiled egg, celery sticks and a little Jarlsberg cheese, chopped together with a few sunflower seeds and a few drops of vinegar.
- Beans on toast with added cherry tomatoes and paprika.
- Soup (home-cooked or ready-made) with crusty bread, watercress and Edam cheese.
- A bagel with low-fat cream cheese, black pepper and wild salmon.
- Low-fat hummus with olives, baby spinach or dandelion leaves and grilled peppers.

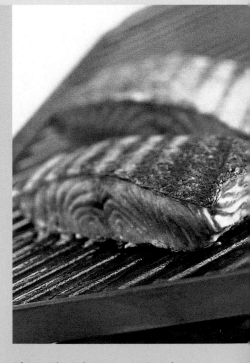

Above Though you're cutting down on fat, make room for plenty of oily fish such as organic salmon. Not only is it a healthy food, its firming, rejuvenating effects on skin far outweigh its calorie count.

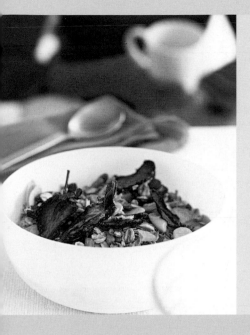

FOODS THAT FIGHT CRAVINGS

Have plenty of the following in your everyday diet, rather than taking supplements that may disrupt your nutritional balance.

Chromium This regulates blood-sugar levels and is found in wholegrain cereals, black pepper, thyme, organic meat and cheese.

Magnesium Found in meats, green leafy vegetables, dairy products, beans, apricots, curry powder, wholegrain cereals, wheatgerm and nuts.

Iron Iron from red meat (especially liver) is most easily used by the body; other good sources are fish and soya, and you can get some from eggs and green leafy vegetables.

Zinc Rich sources are wholegrains, brewer's yeast, wheatgerm, seafood and meat.

Tryptophan Milk and eggs contain plenty of this amino acid.

Above Replace the cloying taste of sugary breakfast cereals with the freshness of fruit, chopped and sprinkled over a mixture of natural grains. For more variety, add some seeds, wheatgerm or nuts.

dinner

Select one of the following ideas, adding as many extra vegetables as you like (for dessert, have some fruit):

- Free-range chicken or tofu (bean curd), stir-fried in oil with onions, courgettes, mangetouts, Chinese leaves, ginger, garlic and soy sauce.
- Tuna with lettuce, cucumber and artichoke hearts, dressed with lemon juice and chopped fresh herbs.
- Organic minced beef and/or canned kidney beans, stewed with spring onions, kale, carrots, peas, potatoes and a dash of Worcestershire sauce.
- Steamed cauliflower, broccoli or fennel with grated cheese. Steamed spinach scattered with pumpkin seeds.
- Mackerel fillet with leeks, coriander and microwaved pumpkin.
- Vegetable curry (home-cooked or low-fat ready-made), brown rice.
- Organic liver and onions fried in a teaspoon of oil, with runner beans, lightly steamed Savoy cabbage and mashed parsnips.

snacks

You may choose two from the following snacks each day:

- A handful of nuts and raisins.
- A piece of fruit.
- A slice of toast with yeast extract.
- A small piece of cheese.
- A small pot of natural low-fat yogurt with chopped berries.
- Six almonds.

weeks 2-6: fast fat burning

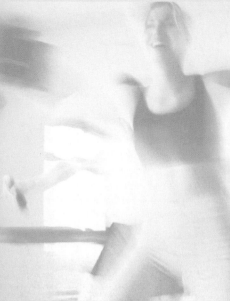

In week 1 you were warming up for this focused exercise regime. The work you've done on stretching and posture should help you exercise more effectively and reduce the risk of injury. The plan from here on is to do three workouts a week, including aerobics, body sculpting and stretching.

For exercise to work, it has to be done regularly. The easiest way to fit exercise into a busy life is to organize your schedule around regular sessions.

Try to do some of your exercise outdoors. Even on a cool day, the fresh air will give you an instant energy boost.

mondays, wednesdays & fridays

Work out at set times on these three days. If you miss a session (which involves aerobics, body sculpting and stretching, see below), fit one in later the same day, or the next morning if you missed an evening workout – but leave at least 24 hours before the next workout. If you can get to a gym, substitute the workout with an aerobics exercise class, and do the body sculpting as a separate session the next day. Best of all, try not to miss any sessions (see box opposite).

Start with 60-minute sessions, which you can increase to 90 minutes from week 3 onwards if you wish:
- **Warm-up** Do a 5-minute warm-up (see page 10).
- **Aerobic exercise** Put on some dance music and do 30–45 minutes aerobic dance, following the instructions on pages 12–13. Slow down over a couple of minutes at the end to bring your heart rate down. Include plenty of Side Swings, Knee Taps and Arm Movements to warm up for the body sculpting and stretches.
- **Body sculpting and stretching** Do 10–20 minutes Super Sculpting (see page 124–125).

the rest of the week

On Tuesdays and Thursdays do a lighter activity, such as a half-hour walk before lunch.
At the weekend do at least an hour's aerobic activity, whether it's playing football with your fiancé, pedalling an exercise bike or going for a swim.

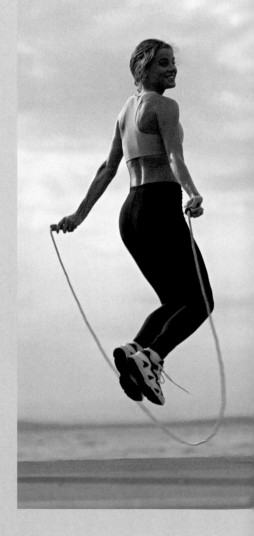

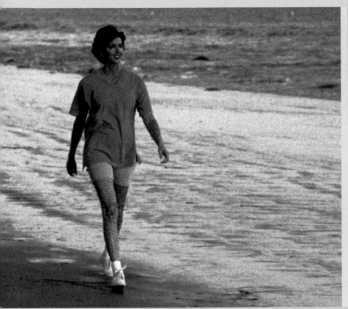

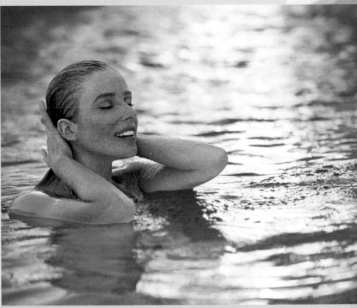

Above Walking on the beach gives your legs a powerful workout as your feet dig into the sand. Then dive in for a swim, enjoying the coolness of water and the effortless grace of weightless movement.

Left Do you think you're as fit as when you were 10 years old? Try a few minutes skipping and see how puffed out you are! No wonder boxers do it. This will soon rebuild your aerobic fitness.

CALORIE BURNING
Being more active is the easiest way to lose weight. You can burn off an extra 90 calories an hour doing the ironing, or 270 calories dancing – it's your choice!

WHEN'S THE BEST TIME TO EXERCISE?
Physically, our bodies are best suited to exercise in the late afternoon. At about 6pm our levels of energy and endurance are at their peak, and we're least likely to have an injury because our muscles are most supple. This fits in with visiting the gym on the way back from work, or working out as soon as you get home. Exercise reduces stress, so it's also effective at shaking off the day's problems.

On the other hand, your plans can easily be derailed by working overtime, your social life or lack of motivation at the end of a day's work. And though regular exercise will help you sleep better, some people find it hard to drop off after an evening workout.

Surveys show that most people who exercise regularly do it in the morning. Not necessarily because they're morning people, but because it's easiest to set the alarm clock early and get it out of the way. It does mean having to exercise without breakfast – or half an hour after a snack of, say, a piece of toast or a few spoonfuls of cereal or yogurt. But you'll burn off every calorie of the big breakfast you've earned afterwards.

The most important thing is to find a time when you can exercise three days a week, and stick to that come what may. Adapting your exercise routine to fit around other commitments may seem a sensible idea, but what tends to happen is that the other things overrun, you miss the exercise slot and hope to fit it in the next day. With your wedding a few weeks off, the next day has its own crowded schedule already. You never quite get time to build up fitness. So, just three times a week, make this your top priority.

weeks 2–6: super sculpting

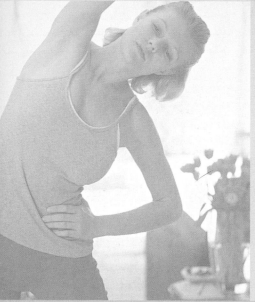

Regular upper-body workouts will enhance the look of most wedding dresses, which reveal your arms and shoulders. Your back, which rarely gets any attention, will be revealed if you wear a strapless dress, and putting your hair up draws more attention to that area. A traditional fitted ballgown also draws attention to your waist. So from week 2 onwards you need to work on these areas, firming your arms and upper body while trimming your waist and building abdominal muscles to hold your stomach in. For best results you'll need a set of weights (see page 39).

how often?

Aim to do 10–20 minutes of body sculpting three times a week, after the aerobic workout described on the preceding pages. (You don't need to warm up for body sculpting if you're doing it straight after aerobics.) From week 3 onwards, you can build up to 30 minutes of body sculpting if you wish.

This Super Sculpting routine focuses on the areas accentuated by most wedding dresses and it's fine to concentrate on those you need most. But to maximize the fat-burning effect of muscle building, do include the Press-Ups and Curl-Ups from page 17.

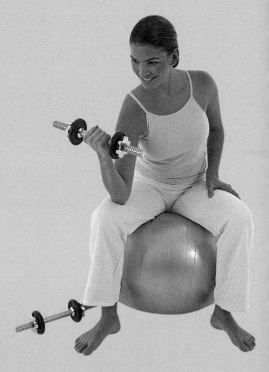

how many?

Do eight repetitions of the following exercises – eight on each side, where relevant – for the first week. After that, work up to two or three sets of 12 reps.

If you want to increase the intensity even further, use the next level of weight, rather than doing yet more repetitions. But if you do this and find you are aching throughout the next day, drop back to the lower weight or fewer reps.

bridal body sculpting

Follow the instructions for the following exercises, which can be found on pages 17 and 38–41.
● Press-Ups: a good all-round exercise for your arms and chest.

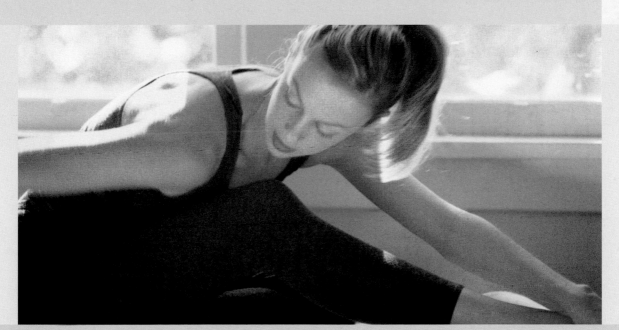

Above Stretching is an essential component of a body-sculpting routine. As well as preventing pain and protecting muscles and joints from injury, it helps create long, sleek curves instead of bulk.

Left To tone and shape muscles, for example with a biceps curl, you need to challenge them. If you're not using body weight (as in a press-up), use a set of weights.

WARM-UPS FOR BODY SCULPTING

If you've substituted an aerobics class for your home workout, do the body sculpting on its own the next day. Start with a warm-up, including plenty of Head and Shoulders exercises and Arm Turns (see page 10), plus the Upper-Body Warm-Up and Stomach and Waist Warm-Up from pages 36–37.

- Curl-Ups: to tone the front abdominal muscle.
- Seated Row: to tone and shape the upper and middle back, and the rear of the shoulders.
- Biceps Curls: for the front of the arms.
- Shoulder Press: to create smooth shoulders.
- Triceps Extension and/or Triceps Dip: for the back of the upper arms – the part most likely to need toning, if you're wearing a sleeveless dress.
- Tension Hold: to strengthen the inner abdominal muscles, to prevent a pot belly.
- Roll-Down: for the abdominal muscles.
- Side Pulses: to work the internal and external oblique muscles to trim the waist.
- Side Bends: the classic waist-whittler.
- Stretching: finish with some long, slow stretches such as those on page 11.

now relax!

This intensive programme shouldn't cause any pain (stop at once if it does), but it may be tiring at first.

To relax after a strenuous workout, lie flat on the floor with your body lengthened, your stomach pushing back towards your spine and your upper body released. Draw your knees up to your chest and hold them with both hands. This will soothe lower-back ache, and also helps if you've hurt your back by pushing an exercise too far. Try circling your knees and rocking slowly from side to side.

index

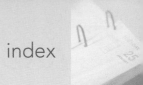

acknowledgements

With thanks to Kate Barlow, Editor of *Wedding* magazine. To subscribe to *Wedding* magazine call 0845 6767778 or click on www.ipcmedia.com

Author acknowledgements

Many thanks to Charles Wenz for endless computer help, and to Marc of Appleaid.net for saving the manuscript. To Lauren and Rog for organizing and to Kath and Tim for dress assistance. To Sue, Vic, Pat, Debbie, Karen, Cora, Richard and all whose efforts contributed to the (in the end) perfect wedding. And above all to David Hall, the perfect bridegroom (he did, as advised, 'wear a suit and turn up') and more importantly the perfect husband.

www.thedietplate.com, tel +44 (0) 1457 862446

Executive Editor
Katy Denny
Editor
Charlotte Wilson
Executive Art Editor
Rozelle Bentheim
Designer
Janis Utton
Senior Production Controller
Martin Croshaw
Picture Researchers
Sophie Delpech
Aruna Mathur